DID YOU EVER SEE A FAT SQUIRREL?

DID YOU EVER SEE A FAT SQUIRREL?

How To Eat Naturally
So You'll Never Be Overweight,
Never Feel Hungry

by Ruth Adams

The paper in this book has been made from waste paper
that normally winds up at the city dump. This reclaimed paper
is an example of how today's wastes can be converted into a
worthwhile resource, thereby helping to solve the solid waste
disposal crisis and preserving the quality of our environment.

RODALE PRESS INC.
EMMAUS, PENNA.   18049

Standard Book Number 0–87857–014–4

Library of Congress Card Number 73–182403

COPYRIGHT 1972

By Ruth Adams

ALL RIGHTS RESERVED

PRINTED IN U.S.A.

B–471

FIRST PRINTING   FEBRUARY 1972

SECOND PRINTING   SEPTEMBER 1974

TABLE OF CONTENTS

The squirrel outside my window this autumn morning bounces over to the dogwood tree where a dozen other squirrels, a cardinal, a towhee, some chickadees are feasting on the mixture of birdseed and sunflower seed I spread around an hour before. After some introductory remarks among the squirrels on who gets first helpings of the sunflower seeds, they all settle down to munching.

This time of year my squirrels are eating mostly seeds and nuts. They have enormous caches of walnuts, butternuts and hickory nuts stored in their tree homes and buried in the ground. They comb through grasses, weeds and leaves for seeds of other kinds, sort them out and carefully put away whatever they do not eat.

In five minutes each squirrel has enough. He leaves, perhaps digging up a buried walnut to carry home. There is still plenty of seed spread on the ground. He's not interested. He's had enough. Why? And why, when he appears to be eating relatively enormous amounts of fat, isn't he fat? I've never seen a fat squirrel living in the wild, eating the food his ancestors have eaten for millions of years. You never saw a fat squirrel living and eating this way. You never saw a fat chickadee or towhee, a fat deer or rabbit living in the wild and eating what their ancestors have eaten through the millions of years that birds and animals have lived on the earth.

Seeds and nuts are the most highly concentrated foods in nature. Meat contains 70 per cent water; apples are 85 per cent water. Seeds and nuts contain very little. They are rich, instead, in protein and fat, with some carbohydrate. Fat? How much fat? Well, almonds are 54 per cent fat, sunflower seeds 47 per cent fat, sesame seeds 49 per cent fat. The walnuts my squirrels eat all winter are 59 per cent fat. And the hickory nuts which are their very favorite foods are 68 per cent fat!

Stand on a street corner in any city in the United States and watch the figures of the people who pass. Count the number you would classify as "overweight," "fat" or "obese." It will amaze you how many there are. Why? When wild animals and birds can so perfectly regulate their eating habits and maintain at all times exactly the right weight for them, even when food is very abundant, how does it happen that we human beings cannot achieve this happy condition?

Does a squirrel have more willpower than we do? Has a squirrel studied nutrition, so he knows which foods to eat and which to ignore? If so, why does he eat so much fat and why doesn't it make him fat? Do squirrels count calories?

The answer to these questions has to do, I believe, with evolution and technology—a far cry from the kind of thing most books on reducing talk about. Squirrels and other wild animals are still eating as they and their ancestors have eaten for millions of years. Human beings in the Western world are eating, instead, large amounts of something called food presented to us as wholesome and nourishing, but differing in so many elementary ways from the food mankind has eaten down through the ages of evolution, that we are totally unable to adapt to it, within the short space of 30 to 50 years, which is all the time we have had.

This book is about addiction, for the giant food industry has produced a large body of addicts among the American people—who cannot get along without their daily drugs—in this case, the refined and processed goodies which food technologists have developed, and which the powerful advertising industry hoodwinks us into buying. Food and the way it is presented to us has suffered from our modern technological revolution perhaps more than any other element in the environment.

The solution to our nutrition problems which is being ever more subtly and cautiously approached by nutrition experts is the same solution we are told by many philosophers will be the only possible solution for most future technological problems. The intellectual elite, the "experts" in any given field will make the decisions and the rest of us will follow meekly along, doing what we are told, uncomprehending and helpless, totally dependent upon the superior knowledge of the specialists in all these complex fields.

In the case of food, a prominent nutrition expert recently bemoaned the fact that just about the entire American population should be put on "special diets." Hardening of the arteries, obesity, high blood pressure, diabetes, tooth decay, various allergies, osteoporosis, gout, kidney disorders, inherited and congenital diseases of metabolism, lack of ability to absorb food and other digestive and eliminative complaints afflict almost the entire population.

This expert, Dr. Mark Hegsted of Harvard University, sees as the only answer a consulting dietician service in supermarkets to which the sick person (and he believes this includes most of us) would bring his doctor's prescription for a diet. The dietician would make out a list of allowed foods *and then the supermarket would sell the customer only those foods he is permitted to eat!* "If the patient continued the service," he says, "it might be difficult not to follow the diet prescribed."

If you think this suggestion is far-fetched in the middle of the 20th century when we are all presumably free agents, there is an excellent example of this kind of thinking already upon us. Tooth decay is one of the near-universal disorders Dr. Hegsted mentions. The causes of tooth decay are well-known. Tooth decay can be, and is, induced at will in laboratory animals by feeding them a "cariogenic" diet which is very much like the diet most of our children eat—a diet in which refined carbohydrates are abundant, especially those which tend to stick around the teeth and remain in the mouth for considerable periods of time. Feeble efforts by doctors and dentists to convey this information on the relation of tooth decay and diet are made from time to time, mostly in words like "limit between-meal sweets" which flash on the TV screen for a second or so.

Since this so-called "nutritional education" has obviously failed, fluoridation of water supplies is presented by the experts as the only practical answer to tooth decay. We are told, time and again, by the dental and public health experts that we—the common or garden variety of human being— simply don't have the know-how to decide for ourselves how to fight tooth decay most effectively. Most of us, we are told, are not even capable of giving our children fluoride tablets, if we feel they should have them to prevent tooth decay.

Nobody tells a squirrel what to eat. Rabbits know their natural food is mostly green, leafy things. Chickadees and goldfinches search out sunflower seeds, while robins hop, cheerful and unconcerned, across our lawns, devouring worms. None of them ever eats too much. None of them ever has a problem with overweight.

It is the theme of this book that we should take our nutrition lessons from these experts. It is the theme of this book that, if we return almost entirely to the kind of food our ancestors ate for all the millions of years of prehistoric times and recorded history, we will also have no desire to overeat and we can free ourselves from our preposterous national burden of overweight and many of the myriad disorders that accompany it.

CHAPTER ONE

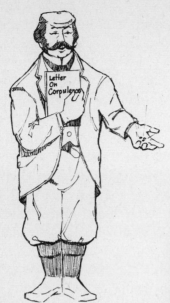

REVERENCE
AND GOLDEN
PIPPINS

WILLIAM BANTING was a formerly fat man who, in 1865, published a little book called *Letter on Corpulence*. He sold 58,000 copies of it. The book told the story of how Mr. Banting lost about one pound a week for 38 weeks and most of the symptoms of ill-health that had plagued him for years. He was so enthusiastic about the diet by which he accomplished all this that he became a resolute crusader and probably bored his overweight friends and acquaintances with relentless urging to follow his example.

He said, in *Letter on Corpulence*,

"Of all the parasites that affect humanity, I do not know of, nor can I imagine any more distressing than that of obesity, and having just emerged from a very long probation in this affliction, I am desirous of circulating my humble knowledge and experience for the benefit of my fellow man, with an earnest hope it may lead to the same comfort and

1

happiness I now feel under the extraordinary change—which might almost be termed miraculous had it not been accomplished by the most simple common sense means. . . . I am very much better, bodily and mentally, and pleased to believe that I hold the reins of health and comfort in my own hands." He took off 35 pounds in 38 weeks. He lost all symptoms of indigestion. He discarded his knee bandages and a truss which he had worn for 20 years.

"The remedy may be as old as the hills, as I have since been told," says Mr. Banting, but that doesn't make it any the less effective. He goes on to say, "I can now confidently say that *quantity* of the diet may be safely left to the natural appetite; and that it is the quality only, which is essential to abate and cure corpulence."

The diet on which this ardent weight watcher lost so much weight consisted of four meals a day, plus a nightcap. He cheerfully discloses just what each meal consisted of. Listen!

For breakfast, four or five ounces of beef, mutton, kidneys, broiled fish, bacon or cold meat of any kind except pork. A large cup of tea with no milk or sugar, plus "a little biscuit" or one ounce of dry toast. This was eaten at 8 to 9 a.m.

For dinner at 1–2 p.m. Mr. Banting took five or six ounces of any meat but pork, any vegetable except potatoes, one ounce of dry toast, "fruit out of a pudding" by which we suppose he meant raw or stewed fruit, any kind of poultry or game, plus two or three glasses of good claret, sherry or "maderia." Champagne, port and beer were forbidden.

For the sacred British institution of tea he had, around 5 or 6 p.m. two or three ounces of fruit, a rusk or two and a cup of tea.

For supper at nine o'clock he ate substantially the

same thing as dinner, with three or four ounces of meat or fish, plus a glass or two of claret.

And at bedtime he had "if required," a tumbler of grog—gin, whiskey or brandy, without sugar, or a glass or two of claret or sherry. We do not know what is meant by a "tumbler." Was it an ounce or was it more?

The modern dieter, accustomed to black coffee for breakfast, cottage cheese for lunch and a lamb chop for dinner will most probably not believe that Mr. Banting ate all this and lost about a pound a week for 35 weeks. But there is medical confirmation for his statements. His doctor who is believed to be Dr. William Harvey, an eye, ear, nose and throat surgeon to the Royal Dispensary, for diseases of the ear, believed that, since food of animal origin was recommended for diabetics because it reduced the sugar in urine, perhaps the same kind of food might do well for obese people, since they might have some of the same characteristics as diabetics.

Dr. Harvey counselled Mr. Banting against eating vegetables that grow below the ground because, said he, "vegetable roots hold a large quantity of saccharine matter" but only beneficial effects come from those vegetables "the fruits of which are on the exterior of the earth, as they lose, probably by means of the sun's action, a large proportion of their sugar."

Without any food lists from the Department of Agriculture to guide him, Dr. Harvey knew that the leaves and stalks of vegetables are rich in some valuable nutrients, but poor in starches and sugars, while vegetables that grow below the surface of the earth, like potatoes, turnips, beets, carrots contain more starch.

From the way he speaks, Mr. Banting had previously been

eating quite large amounts of sugar as well as bread, for which, he says, he always had a great fondness. He took sugar with his tea and had pastries and tarts for dinner and supper. He drank lots of beer. And one surmises that he was accustomed to adding sugar to wine, since he points out in his new diet recommendations that this must never be done. It sounds almost unbelievable, but, after he went on his diet, *he found that by adding only one ounce of sugar a day (two tablespoons) he increased his weight by one pound in only seven days! This is the power of sugar in adding weight!*

We don't know why his doctor forbade pork which is excellent food, or salmon which, we know today contains the valuable unsaturated fats. Nor do we know why he allowed sherry but forbade port, since these two wines today contain about the same amount of sugar. Perhaps they were made differently a hundred years ago.

Vitamins were unknown in those days. Today we know that a diet like the one Mr. Banting followed might present problems for someone with rather high requirements for several vitamins. Unless Mr. Banting went out of his way to eat rather large amounts of deep green and bright yellow vegetables and citrus fruits, he might have had difficulty getting enough vitamin A and vitamin C for good health. If he ate liver several times a week, this would take care of the vitamin A requirement. But a modern dieter would do well to assure himself of ample vitamins by taking care to get lots of the brightly-colored green and yellow vegetables as well as popping an all-round vitamin pill into his mouth every morning at breakfast.

Did the fat people of the world welcome Mr. Banting's experience and fly to emulate him? Apparently he managed to convert some close friends to his way of eating. But the world in general, and the world of orthodox medicine in particular scorned his book, disbelieved his testimony and went right on saying that it's a well known scientific fact that, to lose weight, you simply have to eat less. It doesn't much matter what you eat, so long as you eat less. Calories do count!

It didn't seem to occur to anybody that Mr. Banting's doctor was experimenting with a whole new theory of nutrition. The theory is that, if your food properly nourishes you, you have no desire to overeat. Meat, vegetables and fruit are foods which we eat in their natural state, except for cooking them. We don't eat too much because our human bodies have been geared to this kind of food for hundreds of thousands of years. We don't overeat on this kind of food any more than a wild squirrel overeats on the nuts and seeds which *his* ancestors have been eating for millions of years.

But add some considerable amounts of sugar and some refined flour—both foods which are of quite recent origin from the point of view of evolution, and you have a different situation entirely. There's no built-in protection against eating too much. And by the time you have baked the sugar and the flour into tarts and pastries, any resemblance to ancestral food has long since disappeared.

Today in metabolic laboratories equipped with unimaginably complex machinery for testing, weighing and estimating, modern nutrition experts treat Mr. Banting's book with a great deal of condescension. They appear to feel that what worked perfectly for him a hundred years ago has little or no relevance to all the fat people alive today—and they number in the millions.

It is the point of view of the writer of this book that Mr. Banting had something, that Mr. Banting made a discovery that is just as valid today as it was a hundred years ago, and that by adapting the diet that worked his miracle to present-day conditions, we can learn not just how to take off pounds, but can learn a whole new way of eating and living, can learn how to thread our way healthfully through the treacherous aisles of the supermarket and the heavily-laden tables of the gourmet restaurant. For the general idea behind Mr. Banting's diet has been shown to be sound by a great many researchers in our modern world. It is to these men that we will turn for confirmation.

The kindly Mr. Banting believed that everyone should adopt his well-tested diet. Then, said he, all the disorders which had plagued him for so long, would become rare indeed, "like reverence and Golden Pippins."

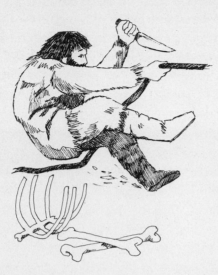

CHAPTER TWO

THE "STONE AGE DIET"

THE ARCTIC EXPLORER, Vilhjalmur Stefansson, was profoundly interested in diet. He lived for years at a time on nothing but fat and lean meat, on his journeys to the Far North. He suffered no harm from such a diet.

After he returned, he got into a mighty scrimmage on the subject of diet. It began with an article of his which was published in the *Journal of the American Medical Association* in 1918. His theory was simply that a diet of nothing but protein and fat was perfectly healthful so long as some of the meat was sufficiently undercooked to leave a little vitamin C there.

In 1926 another *JAMA* article by Dr. Clarence Lieb discussed Stefansson's diet, described his own examination of the explorer and stated that he was in a state of health equal to, or better than, that of the average man. When the American Meat Institute became interested, the explorer found himself involved in a scientific experiment which should, he believed, give an unequivocal answer to the arguments about the wholesomeness of an all-meat diet.

Arrangements were made for a 13-month test at Bellevue Hospital, with the diets of Stefansson and another volunteer carefully supervised, weighed and assayed for fat and lean content. For the first six months, the explorer and his friend both lived at the hospital. There seems to be no doubt among even the most skeptical observers that Stefansson and his friend lived exactly as they had undertaken to live throughout these months. There was no cheating. Nobody slipped anything sweet or starchy into them at the hospital, although they were supposedly craving this kind of food.

According to Stefansson, they hankered for none of the forbidden goodies. He tells us that if they ever got hungry it was always for more meat. And since they were allowed in this test to have as much meat as they wished, they simply ate more meat whenever they wanted it. They ate lean and fat meat. They took in a daily average of about 2600 to 2800 calories, practically all of it derived from protein and fat, since meat contains almost no carbohydrate.

They ate nothing else at all. They did not even go out of their way to eat the especially nutritious organ meats like liver and kidneys. As summer approached critics who had predicted catastrophe from the beginning, foretold the end of the test when hot weather struck. They claimed it was a well known scientific fact that meat in the diet creates heat in the body, and someone living on an exclusive meat diet could not possibly survive hot weather.

It was an especially hot summer, says Stefansson. Neither he nor his colleague experienced the slightest discomfort due to heat.

By the end of the test they were both in as good condition

as they had been when they started. They had been careful to go through an initial period on the usual mixed diet during which time they were tested by experts in all kinds of ways. At the end of the experiment they once again were subjected to tests. Then they went into another several weeks of mixed diet and further tests were given. It was the medical consensus that they were both in as good condition as they had been at the beginning of the experiment which had lasted for 13 months. Perhaps they were in even better condition.

Blood sugar levels had to be reoriented at the end of the test. Or, more simply, the glands which regulate blood sugar levels had to become accustomed once again to working with the additional sugar and starch which were involved when desserts, cereals, fruits and vegetables were once again included in their meals.

Such an experiment, carried on for more than a year, speaks volumes for the dedication and conviction of Stefansson who was trying to prove something very basic about the nutrition of man. As an authority on life in the Far North, he had to show doubting Thomases, he thought, that men could live in excellent health and also be content eating nothing but protein and fat. As an Arctic expert, he was called on many times for advice in equipping and feeding expeditions of one kind or another. If he did not convince the experts that fat and lean meat make a complete, wholly healthful diet, how could he advise them what food to take along for Arctic living?

But, aside from this, Stefansson was a remarkable man with a vast range of interests. Nutrition was one of them. Almost alone among men with a nutritional theory, he proved his theory on himself, by living, as he had predicted he could, on the diet which others warned him might be fatal. According to him, there was no inconvenience so far as the diet was concerned. That is, he had no difficulty "getting used" to it. He had no pangs, no cravings for forbidden foods, no feelings of deprivation.

Yet the very bother of subjecting himself to constant testing, and confining himself to New York during most of the experiment must have tested severely the patience and forbearance of a man whose interests were so wide, for all his activities necessarily had to be curtailed that entire year— not because the diet was in the least hard to come by, but because he had to report in, and be available for conferences, tests and affirmations, so that no critic could ever be able to say the test had not been a fair one.

Considering the hardships of such dedication, then, it is discouraging that present-day nutrition science—the official part of it, that is—almost completely ignores the theory proven so laboriously by Stefansson that fat and protein make a complete diet. In fact whenever it is suggested that a diet consisting almost exclusively of protein and fat is a good diet, hands still go up in horror, voices are still raised in condemnation. We, the long suffering public, are still told, "it's a well known scientific fact" that man cannot live on fat and protein alone, that eating fat will cause one to put on weight, for calories *do* count and the important thing to remember is that you can keep your weight down *only* by restricting calories to such and such an amount. If you want to use up all those calories on starch and sugar, this is perhaps not the wisest thing to do, no, but it's possible to reduce this way! That's what the authorities are saying, in essence.

Stefansson took no more than his usual exercise while he was on his all-meat diet. For all his many activities, he must have spent much of his time in conferences, writing or reading—very sedentary occupations. By actual measurement, he was eating up to 2800 calories a day, *80 per cent of these calories coming from fat meat. He did not put on any weight.*

Something more. He did not feel hungry. He did not suffer the agonies of today's fatties trying to get along on dry toast and coffee for breakfast and a dab of cottage cheese for lunch. His breakfast of fat and lean meat—fat and protein—kept him content until lunch. His lunch of additional fat and protein kept him well satisfied until dinner time. So his diet overcame the chief drawback to most reducing diets—the hunger that accompanies them.

Whether you overeat out of emotional need, or for status, or to spite somebody, or because you just don't have any guts, you'll have to admit that it's hard, very hard, to force oneself to overeat if one just isn't hungry. And when one has just finished a meal consisting of 80 per cent fat it's understandable that one would find it hard to eat more fat. There is a satiety value to fat. You simply get nauseated if you happen to eat too much by mistake.

Today, high protein diets do not consist exclusively of meat. They would be too expensive, for one thing. The job of tapering off from a diet high in carbohydrates to one in which they are almost eliminated could be upsetting for someone who knows little about nutritional needs. Today a diet rich in protein, with plenty of low carbohydrate fruits and vegetables for variety, can produce the same results Stefansson had for less money and less inconvenience. This is the diet this book recommends.

11

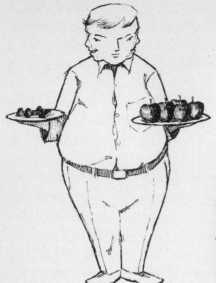

CHAPTER THREE

DR. CLEAVE AND THE SACCHARINE DISEASE

D R. T. L. CLEAVE, of Hants, England, a Surgeon Captain in the Royal Navy, bases his thinking about obesity and a surprising number of other diseases, on Darwin's theory of evolution. Man, along with animals, has adapted himself to his environment in order to survive. Disease (including obesity) occurs because of some hereditary defect *or because of some new element in the environment*.

In a book entitled *Diabetes, Coronary Thrombosis and the Saccharine Disease*, which he co-authored in 1966 with Dr. G. D. Campbell, he says "If the disease is due to hereditary defect—that is, the body is built wrongly—the only treatment possible will be either operative repair or some form of replacement therapy: whereas if the disease is due to a new factor in the environment—that is, the body is being used wrongly—the treatment is at once directed to the removal of the cause. The two types of treatment are poles apart."

The "new factor" in the environment which, according to this theory, is the cause of much of our modern disease, is the refinement and sophistication of our food, something which has occurred only within the past 50 years or so in the history of Western civilization and, with great new intensity, only within the past 25 years.

In refining cereals and sugarcane, we remove certain parts of the original foods. From wheat, for instance, we take most of the germ and most of the bran or outer coat. Sugarcane is a fibrous stalk of which our refineries discard everything except the sugar itself. In each case, we have concentrated certain parts of the food, discarding the rest.

This concentration, says Dr. Cleave, *which is a very recent development in terms of human history,* deceives the tongue and the appetite and leads to overconsumption, "and this overconsumption is the sole primary cause of the overweight. With unrefined, unconcentrated carbohydrates over-consumption does not occur, and obesity does not occur, either, as we intend to demonstrate."

He goes on to say that this theory excludes as a primary cause of obesity any fault in the instinct of appetite or any lack of exercise. "In short, it is advanced that, as regards obesity, the body, again, is not built wrongly, but is being used wrongly."

Say Drs. Cleave and Campbell in their *Saccharine Disease,* "A glance at any wild creature in its natural environment shows that no matter how plentiful its food supply, it never eats too much of it. . . . no wild rabbit ever ate too much grass, no wood-pigeon ever ate too much wheat, and no herring ever ate too much plankton. No wild creature, in fact, is ever overweight.* The forces of evolution have en-

---

* It is well known that some wild animals carry considerable weight for some sound physiological reason: hibernation, warmth, buoyancy. This is not pathological overweight.

sured that in nature organisms react to an abundant food supply never by developing a disease, such as obesity, but by raising the rate at which they propagate themselves. This is true for the whole of creation, from a lactic acid bacillus in a bottle of milk right up to man himself in circumstances of plenty. . . . we intend to show that the freedom from obesity in organisms living under natural conditions applies equally to, for example, Africans still living in a tribal manner on unrefined foods."

"It is therefore contended," they go on, "that the *sole* cause of obesity lies in the consumption of refined carbohydrates. . . . Equally it should be thoroughly realized that unrefined carbohydrates such as wholemeal bread, potatoes eaten in their skins, raw fruit, and so forth, are no more fattening than any other natural food, including protein foods and fatty foods."

Dr. Campbell's observations on members of the Zulu tribe in South Africa are then detailed. Other observations by other workers seem to show exactly the same thing. Urban Zulus, able to buy "white man's food," show about the same proportion of overweight individuals as there are in America. Those Zulus still living in the country and unable to get any appreciable amount of refined food, are remarkably free from obesity, *in spite of the fact that 90 per cent of their calories come from carbohydrate foods, as against 81 per cent carbohydrate in the urban food of the urban Zulus.*

This is another proof, according to Dr. Cleave, that carbohydrates per se are not responsible for overweight. Eaten in their natural state, they do not result in overeating. It is only when they are refined and concentrated that our tongues and appetites can no longer deal with them nor estimate successfully how much we should eat of carbohydrate food. That is the reason we overeat.

14

"The appetite is not regarded as an enemy here, to be placed in a strait jacket, but as a normal instinct, to be let loose on foods so naturally diluted by fibre that the instinct is neutralized in a natural manner," say Drs. Cleave and Campbell.

In an earlier book on *Peptic Ulcer* Dr. Cleave has simplified his argument still further by comparing a fair-sized unpeeled apple to a piece of chocolate. The apple contains the same number of calories you might find in a very small piece of chocolate. You can eat perhaps five pieces of chocolate at once. Could you possibly eat five apples at one time?

The average person in Great Britain, which is where Dr. Cleave lives and writes, eats 5 ounces of sugar a day. This much sugar is extracted from two and a half pounds of sugar cane, or sugar beets. Who could eat that much of the original food every day? "In the refining of carbohydrates," says Dr. Cleave, "the refining processes lead to increased consumption. It would seem that this is due to the fact that the unnatural concentration deceives the taste-buds in the tongue."

Then, too, the removal of fiber reduces the time it takes for these foods to pass through the stomach. So, quite apart from blood sugar considerations, one is hungry sooner after eating refined sugar or a white flour product than if he has consumed an apple or some other piece of fruit, or a piece of real whole grain bread. If you've never tasted the latter— and very few modern Americans ever have—it's tough, hard to chew. And it stays with you!

Dr. Cleave relates the refining of food to the entire group of disorders which he calls "The Saccharine Disease." This has nothing to do with the artificial sweetener, saccharin. Instead it refers to modern refined sugar and the starch in white flour and commercial cereals which is converted to

15

sugar in the body. His arguments are most persuasive, for he buttresses them with convincing statistics on the incidence of obesity, diabetes, coronary thrombosis, ulcer and varicose veins in populations which consume large amounts of refined carbohydrates compared to those populations where such foods are unknown.

In vain have critics of Dr. Cleave's theory tried to demolish it with quibbling and nit-picking. One critic wrote furiously to the *British Medical Journal* that he just couldn't be right about the absence of varicose veins in native, rural Africans. Why, said he, you just can't see the varicose veins because the women wear long skirts and besides they don't show as clearly on dark-skinned people.

Dr. Cleave whipped back a speedy answer quoting careful surveys made in hospitals where Africans are cared for and hospitals where Americans, both white and black, are cared for. One African hospital reports only five cases of varicose veins among more than 14,000 admissions. In Western nations, including the USA, varicose veins are believed to affect about 10 per cent of our population! This would be 2,000,000 people. Presumably the percentage among hospital patients would be even higher since many of them are there for operations on varicose veins.

Perhaps talk about varicose veins has no place in a book on overweight. But perhaps it has. If indeed, as Dr. Cleave postulates, all these disorders spring from one basic cause, perhaps you may have many more premiums than just reducing, if you decide to follow the diet which he recommends to his patients. Wouldn't it be nice to avoid varicose veins, as well, to say nothing of heart attacks, diabetes, peptic ulcer and hemorrhoids?

Dr. Cleave's diet sheet follows at the end of this chapter.

We have omitted most of his remarks on various diseases other than obesity. And we have translated certain very British expressions into Americanese for easier understanding.

Of course in any congregation of scientists, each with his own theory to defend, his own place in the hierarchy to maintain, perhaps his own financial grant to justify, there is always somebody who comes up with the argument that people in Western countries have plumbing and television sets and people in rural Africa don't, so therefore, this chap argues, there is just as much reason to say that plumbing and TV are the cause of overweight as there is to say that it's caused by refined flour and sugar. People who argue like this generally manage to get out of the room before you have time to point out to them that somehow when the rural Africans move into town, they still can't afford TV or plumbing, but their weight begins to increase as soon as they have access to candy, soft drinks, bakery products and so forth, and as soon as they begin to substitute these for most of the natural foods their ancestors have been eating for thousands of years.

There are, too—and it grieves us to record this—university scientists in the field of nutrition who try to demolish theories like Dr. Cleave's by pointing out that he doesn't ask us to eat the shells of nuts, or the straw of the wheat, or all the branches and leaves of a fruit tree—so how then can he say he is in favor of only "whole foods." Aren't we "diluting foods" when we remove the shell from the walnut, they ask. Aren't we "diluting foods" when we eat only the head of the cabbage and throw away the stalk?

This is a specious argument and the nutrition experts who use it know that it is specious, but they continue to use it

17

because it throws some confusion into the controversy and alienates a lot of people who might otherwise be interested in Dr. Cleave's position.

So far as we know, mankind is unequipped by nature to eat the shells of nuts or the branches of trees. For perhaps 10,000 years—since the discovery of ways to plant and harvest cereals, he has been eating the head of the cereal—that is, just the part in which the seed is contained. He has always discarded the stalk, probably because he could find no way to pulverize it sufficiently to make it edible. It is Dr. Cleave's contention that in these 10,000 years men have become adapted to cereals as food—whole cereals, that is. Whole because there was in the past no way to make them anything but whole.

Quite recently in history enterprising technologists discovered how to mill grains in such a way that the tough chewy part is removed and the flour comes out fine as face powder and chalky white after it is bleached. To achieve this, as we have stated above, the germ and the bran are almost entirely removed. We have white flour. Until perhaps 100 years ago white flour was a delicacy available only to the very rich in most parts of the Western world. It is only within the past 25 or 50 years that white flour products have become dirt cheap and available everywhere in the Western world.

Now there is quite a difference, from the point of view of evolution, between 10,000 years and 50 years. Dr. Cleave is contending simply that the human body has not had time to adjust to this drastic change in its one staple, basic food, the Staff of Life. Whether another 10,000 years might bring about such an adaptation remains to be seen. None of us will be around to report. But our present enormous and almost universal (in terms of the "civilized" world) problem

18

with overweight stems entirely, says Dr. Cleave, from this attempt to by-pass the evolutionary process and make highly concentrated foods the basis of our menus when our bodies have not had a period of many thousands of years to adapt to such food.

The Saccharine Disease was reviewed in the *British Medical Journal,* July 16, 1966, by Derrick Dunlop who said, in part, "That the excessive consumption of refined carbohydrates is the main nutritional error in this country and in most others would be generally agreed; many of us think it far more deleterious than the excessive consumption of animal fats. Further, it is generally agreed to be one of the important factors in the causation of diabetes, dental caries, and obesity. . . . It (Dr. Cleave's theory) seems too simple a theory to be true, but . . . it would be unwise to dismiss it solely on this ground, and were it indeed true the authors have made a bigger contribution to medicine than most university departments make in a generation. The book infuriates but is exciting, interesting and thoughtful."

Few American nutrition experts or MD's appear to have heard of Dr. Cleave. This is not surprising. They know little of most of the information in this book. I could not find a review of any of Dr. Cleave's books in American medical literature. He is treated with great respect in England.

A review of his earlier book, *Peptic Ulcer,* in the *British Medical Journal,* January 26, 1963 said, in part, "The first objection that can be made to this thesis is that the author's argument takes the form of special pleading, because he has gathered together a large collection of miscellaneous data which can be used to support his contention without making an adequate examination of other possibilities. However, before dismissing this type of approach we must remember that it was repeatedly employed by Darwin, who remains one of the giants of biology. . . . though I cannot believe that the author advances anything approaching scientific proof for his views, I nevertheless read his monograph with interest and pleasure and I think that it will be enjoyed by many other physicians."

Here are the general precepts of Dr. Cleave's diet. White flour must be replaced by real wholemeal flour. Any dish involving white rice or any other processed cereal must be fortified, that is, made more "whole" by adding to it some unprocessed bran, thus restoring the fiber and much of the nutrient of the original cereal. For sugar, substitute fruits—but not the dried ones, for they are far too rich in sugar.

Avoid eating "ready-mixed" foods, says Dr. Cleave, for if you eat foods separately by themselves (he gives the examples of boiled eggs, bread, butter and even a little sweetened tea) *you will eat only what you want of each food.* But if the eggs, flour, butter and sugar have been mixed up into a cake, the proportions may not be at all what you may happen to want or have an appetite for. They will be selected according to what proportions result in the best cake from the point of view of the cook!

By the same token, eating fried foods gets you involved in eating a great deal of fat that you may not be hungry for at all, just so that you can have the potatoes or whatever else was fried. "The closer food is to the natural state and the less it is cooked up, the better," says Dr. Cleave. Avoid those foods which stimulate acid secretion by the stomach without neutralizing any of it. Here he mentions coffee and alcohol—most to be avoided by those who suffer from indigestion and ulcer and he adds, "They are at their most dangerous when taken by themselves." (Take heed, all you plump ones, who have been trying to reduce on black coffee and nothing much else!)

20

If you find yourself constipated when you begin his diet, Dr. Cleave recommends bran—plain, unprocessed bran which you will probably have to get at a health food store in this country. Take a teaspoon before meals, washed down with some fluid. Increase the dose if you must, gradually.

Finally, the transition to the recommended diet must be made slowly, *so as at all times to keep in step with the appetite*—that is, with the liking for the natural foods indicated. Follow the natural instinct of appetite, as long as it is allowed to play on natural foods. "Eating natural foods that you do not desire will achieve very little; and eating unnatural foods that you do desire will achieve infinitely less," says Dr. Cleave.

And he ends his homily with this thought, "People are prepared to take endless trouble over the maintenance of a motor car, but over the maintenance of that infinitely more delicate mechanism, the human body, they are seldom prepared to take any trouble at all."

Dr. Cleave's other books are listed in the bibliography at the end of this book. We enthusiastically recommend them all.

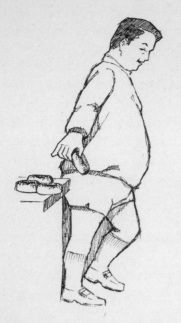

CHAPTER FOUR

IF YOU ARE A SUGAR ADDICT YOU SHOULD REALLY MAKE AN EFFORT

AT QUEEN ELIZABETH COLLEGE, University of London, England, the Professor of Nutrition and Dietetics, John Yudkin, who has both a Ph.D. and an M.D. degree, has some revolutionary ideas on nutrition and health. Like Dr. Cleave, he engages in brisk, lively encounters with other specialists, in the pages of medical and scientific journals. He is a leading spokesman for good, common sense in nutrition. He bulwarks his trenchant attacks on well-established ideas on reducing with ample documentation. He deals not only with nutrition in relation to obesity, but also in relation to coronary heart disease, diabetes and other disorders which apparently are related to diet.

He said in part, at the Symposium on Carbohydrates and Nutrition of the Nutrition Society, "It is generally held that, for the greater part of the million or more years of his existence, man was a hunter and forager; his diet was largely the bodies of animals he killed or found as carrion, with relatively small amounts of leaves, fruits and roots. Being omnivorous (capable of eating any kind of food) he could of course sustain himself if necessary with a lower proportion of meat, and a higher proportion of vegetable foods, but by and large his diet was relatively poor in carbohydrate.

"With the discovery and development of agriculture some eight thousand or 10 thousand years ago, the ease of production of carbohydrate-rich foods such as cereals resulted in his diet with few exceptions becoming predominantly carbohydrate, with little fat and with small and often minimal amounts of protein."

In the Armstrong Memorial Lecture delivered in February, 1962 he added these thoughts: "The revolution in the *quality* of our diet which came about with the discovery of cereals has . . . been followed much more recently by a revolution in *quantity*. The first change, as we saw, has lasted about 10,000 years, one-hundredth of the period of our existence, as a separate species. The second, quantitative, change has lasted less than a century—less, that is, than one-hundredth of one-hundredth of the period of our existence. The qualitative change in our diet from mainly meat to mainly vegetable we owe to the revolution following the discovery of cereals. The quantitative change from constantly recurring hunger to nearly perpetual satiety we owe to the technological revolution."

Dr. Yudkin goes on to talk about what we actually eat in comparison with what we should eat. He tells the story of a wise researcher, Dr. Clara Davis, who found that infants left from six months of age on to choose their own food from a wide selection soon began to eat exactly those foods which were most nourishing. Over the six years of her experiment, the children grew and developed as well as other

23

children, *although they were permitted to eat anything they wanted and as much as they wanted of the food spread before them at each meal.*

But—and here's the rub—the foods from which they could choose did not include anything made with sugar or flour. They were, in every sense of the word, wholly natural foods. No candy, no soft drinks, no desserts, no ice cream, no jam. The children did not miss these foods. They were perfectly happy and well nourished, while they made their own choices, with no interference from adults, among meat, eggs, fruits, and vegetables.

Dr. Yudkin's quarrel with technology is that it has been able to separate palatability from nutrition. That is, modern food processors can make food that tastes good but does not nourish one. Such a food does not exist in nature, so our taste buds have no experience with it. Seeking the sweet taste our ancestors enjoyed in fruits and berries, we eat sugar. But the fruits and berries contain vitamins and minerals, some protein and plenty of fiber. The sugar is "pure." So a good taste no longer has any relation to nourishment in foods. "I believe," says Dr. Yudkin, "that sugar, and perhaps other foods which are being developed to satisfy our palates rather than our bodily needs, constitute a real and growing danger to the nation's nutritional health."

In a *Lancet* article, June 22, 1963, Dr. Yudkin pursues his theory farther. He says, "It is sometimes supposed that obesity is usually caused by an uncontrollable desire to eat. The fact is that those who cannot keep their carbohydrate-restricted diet have, rather, an uncontrollable desire to eat highly palatable sugar-containing foods, to which they have, it seems, become addicted. Obesity was rarely seen in the Eskimo in his original environment, when he had very little access to carbohydrate-containing foods; it is one of the consequences of the introduction to his diet of sugar, sweet drinks, and flour."

If we are looking for some relation between man's diseases (obesity among them) we should try to find what has changed most in his biological environment in the past centuries. Ten thousand years ago a basic change was made. Man settled down into communities and began to raise most of his food in cultivated fields. His days of wandering and gathering food wherever it might be, were over, for most of us, that is. Civilization, as we call it, with all its political and social organization, began with the introduction of cereal foods. But within the past century—100 years, no more— food technologists have developed the skill to separate almost completely the palatability of foods from their nutritive content. They can (and do) make foods which consist of nothing but sweet taste and calories in the form of "pure" carbohydrate. People who know nothing of nutrition and our need for many different nutriments are easily persuaded to consume such foods in abundance. They taste so good that even when more nutritious foods are available it is pleasant to stuff yourself on these goodies.

"As a result," says Dr. Yudkin, "nutritional deficiency does not disappear and in fact sometimes becomes more common. In the wealthier countries, too. . . . we are seeing the displacement of some of the nutritionally more desirable foods from our diets by the tempting but less desirable foods."

Dr. Yudkin believes, he says, that the rapid rise in the incidence of heart attacks is due in part to changes in work, transportation and leisure, brought about by technology, which make modern man increasingly immobile. The second cause is "the availability of highly palatable foods which he is tempted to eat with no reference to his nutritional needs."

In 1964 Dr. Yudkin wrote a book, *The Complete Slimmer,* incorporating his ideas on a healthful reducing diet. It's an interesting and provocative book—witty, outspoken, down-to-earth. We have never seen it in an American bookstore, so it has escaped the free-for-all controversies that have raged here around many another such book.

Dr. Yudkin believes our bodies have an "appestat"—an appetite regulating device which functions well when we are engaged in enough physical activity, but begins to become disordered when we are not. That's right, people who work fairly hard physically tend to eat less than those who just sit around. And, as the physical fitness experts keep warning us, more and more of us tend to just sit around more and more of the time. The scientific experiments which Dr. Yudkin quotes to illuminate this proposition seem to show quite clearly that the more physical activity you engage in the less you will probably eat, in the long run. So there's no longer any excuse for a fatty to say, "I can't exercise, because exercise makes me hungry and I overeat." It doesn't and you don't.

Speaking of reducing diets, Dr. Yudkin takes up the low-fat kind. You know the kind. Dry toast and black coffee for breakfast. Cottage cheese made from skimmed milk for lunch. Meat with every bit of fat pared off for dinner, salad with nothing but lemon juice for dressing.

He reminds us that fat in your diet makes the food stay in your stomach longer, so if you have some fat at every meal, you don't feel empty and hungry so soon after that meal. Then, too, it seems that people who manage to cut out practically all the fat from their diets become irritable and

26

tire easily. They lack the ability to concentrate, they tend to have bad skins. Most important, perhaps, they are not at all reluctant to give up their diets, since the side effects are so unpleasant.

Cutting down on protein can be downright dangerous, he says. We do not know exactly how much protein the average adult needs. Most experts agree it should be not less than 65 grams a day. In Chapter 10 Dr. Yudkin concludes that reducing fat in the diet does not produce a satisfactory diet for most people, that reducing protein is either difficult or dangerous, *but that we eat far too much carbohydrate.* He reminds us too that many of the foods which are high in carbohydrate are also high in fat, so by eliminating them from meals you can also eliminate many calories from fat. In this chapter he presents very convincing arguments that we are rapidly becoming addicted to sugar. That is the word he uses—*addiction, just like drug addiction.*

In England, he says, the average person currently eats nearly five times more sugar than he did 100 years ago. *Today he eats in only two weeks the same amount of sugar the average Britisher ate in a year two centuries ago!* The same is, of course, true in our country.

Dr. Yudkin suggests that you begin your reducing diet by keeping your carbohydrate allowance to 15 carbohydrate units a day. He defines his carbohydrate unit as one-fifth the amount of carbohydrate in an average serving of food. Applying this method to a typical meal, you might eat a serving of meat that contains no carbohydrate, a serving of potatoes containing three carbohydrate units, a serving of broccoli with no carbohydrate units and an apple with two carbohydrate units. The total of five carbohydrate units is all you have to count. You may eat as much protein and fat with the meal as you wish, without counting.

If you don't lose as much weight as you want to lose in two or three weeks, cut to 10 carbohydrate units a day. Do not try to correlate Dr. Yudkin's CU's with the list of carbohydrate grams in the back of this book. Keep in mind that Dr. Yudkin's CU is equal to five grams of carbohydrate. It seems to me that this is confusing to the average non-mathematical person, so I suggest using my carbohydrate list instead. There are no restrictions on anything else in your diet except carbohydrates. You may eat as much meat as you like, as much salad oil as you like, as much cheese, seafood, milk and eggs as you like. There's no need to keep any count of these foods which are, of course, protein and fat foods containing almost no carbohydrate.

The only time that you must make allowance for them in your CU accounting is when they are prepared with some food that has a CU rating. Eat as much hamburger as you like any time of the day or night. But if you eat it on a bun, chalk up 6 CU's. If you eat it with spaghetti, mark down 10 CU's. Two eggs and bacon for breakfast? Why not? It's only protein and fat. But add a piece of toast—any kind—and it will cost you 3 CU's. If you beat up the two eggs into a plain cake for lunch, you must add 5 CU's to your daily total because of the sugar and flour which are in the cake, of course.

You can eat a whole chicken if you happen to feel so inclined. But just one serving of chicken pie will necessitate adding the piecrust CU's to the daily total. Eat as much cheese as you want with every meal or before bedtime. Who's counting? But spread it on 3 crackers and you're saddled with 3 CU's. With salads you have free rein. Dump a whole can of tuna fish into a bowl and eat it all with gobs of mayonnaise, radishes, celery, coleslaw, lettuce and any other salad fixin's you enjoy. Won't cost you a single CU.

But stay away from the melba toast, the potato chip or the roll if you want to keep your CU total low for the day. A cup of coffee or tea is gratis. One teaspoon of sugar in it adds one CU. Milk is allowed any time—any amount you want. But the moment you slip into it any of the "drinks" that are advertised for flavoring it, start counting.

Dr. Yudkin says, and there seems to be no reason to disbelieve him, that you will eat fewer calories on this kind of diet. Talking about eating a whole chicken doesn't mean you will ever want to. Not only will you be eating far less carbohydrate than you ordinarily eat, on the CU slimming diet, but you will also eat less fat. Dr. Yudkin guarantees it. If you stick to the required number of CU's, that is.

He relates his experiences with some apparent failures. One young man who protested that he had been following the diet religiously and failed to lose in six weeks was asked to go over, with Dr. Yudkin, everything he had eaten during one typical day. He had been told to confine his carbohydrates to 10 CU's a day. But it came out that he had eaten 3 crackers at breakfast, two rolls and a glass of fruit juice at lunch, a cheese cracker at dinner and a glass of Ovaltine at bedtime. The total came to 40 CU's instead of ten!

Anybody can cheat, if he wants to. But he can't take off weight that way. And the incentive for not cheating seems to be high with Dr. Yudkin's diet, for you are never hungry. How could you be hungry? You will never have to feel sorry for yourself or deprived of all the goodies everybody else is eating. At any meal, any time, any place, there is always something you can eat—and you can eat as much of it as you want. The point is *you will not want to overeat,* for the things you will eat will "stay with you" and keep you from toppling over from hunger and faintness.

What about drinking? Is a cocktail party likely to throw

off your whole program? One ounce of whiskey, gin, or other distilled liquor contains only a trace of CU's. Three ounces of dry table wine is 3 CU's. Three ounces of sweet table wine is 4 CU's. So pick your drinks with discretion, mix them with water only and stay away from canapes with crackers underneath. Eat as much as you want of the cheese, the salami, the smoked oysters, radishes, celery, olives and so forth.

Two further words of Dr. Yudkin's are memorable. He says, "We have been getting used to lots of new sorts of foods, especially sweet foods. And gradually we become passionately fond of them. Our social habits involve nibbles and snacks and nips we do not at all need for our nutritional well-being. And, more than any other single thing, we have come to worship 'labour-saving' to the extent of growing increasingly immobile. All of these things, and many others, knock sideways the appestat, the controlling mechanism which should see that we eat only as much as we need. Tempting foods or worry or social habit make us eat when we do not need to eat. And inactivity reduces our need for food to a point where the appestat just can't work properly. . . . .

"The fact is that most overweight people are eating not only too much food but also the wrong food. So you have to teach yourself not only to eat less but to eat better. Put another way round, a sensible slimming diet will probably be more nutritious than your ordinary way of eating, even though it will be less food."

Dr. Yudkin's *Complete Slimmer* concludes with a list of common foods and their carbohydrate units. Unfortunately this list is geared to the needs of Englishmen. Many foods listed are unknown in this country, or are known by other names. Many of our favorite foods (and trickiest from the point of view of dieting) are unknown apparently in England. Pizza, for instance, and lasagna, casseroles and many different kinds of sweets. But you can make your own list of foods along with their Carbohydrate Units, if you want to follow Dr. Yudkin's diet completely. It will be easier, perhaps, to follow instead the recommendations we make which are exactly the same, differing only from the point of view of mathematics and how you figure carbohydrate.

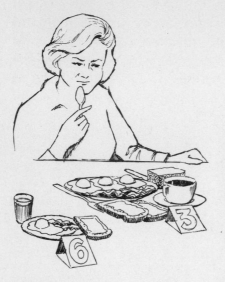

CHAPTER FIVE

WHAT HAS LOW BLOOD SUGAR TO DO WITH LOSING WEIGHT?

"**O**BESITY, even when it results from overeating, is not simply a matter of gluttony or emotional disorder. At the New York Academy of Sciences Conference on Adipose Tissue Metabolism and Obesity, evidence was presented that many obese individuals suffer from an excess of circulating insulin, which lowers blood sugar and causes hunger. . . . this also increases the genesis and storage of fat and impairs carbohydrate metabolism." We are quoting from *Medical World News* for February 5, 1965. This news magazine is edited by the man who was editor of the *Journal of the American Medical Association* for many years.

Here is a story from *New Scientist,* an English publication, which also appeared in the *Journal of the American Medical Association.* It concerns the work of Dr. E. S. Gordon of the University of Wisconsin who found out that one way to help people to lose weight was to feed them six small meals a day, rather than the three which some of us eat, or the two, or even one which apparently quite a few of us have been eating for years.

Dr. Gordon injected a radioactive form of sugar to see what happened to it in his obese patients. He found that the fatties use the sugar chiefly for storing fat, rather than for manufacturing energy. "According to Dr. Gordon this is the basic metabolic defect causing obesity, and overweight people may actually eat no more carbohydrate than the average person."

A great deal of work has, of necessity, been done on the body's use of sugar and what happens to the sugar in one's blood as a result of different diets. One reason for this is that we have a large and increasing number of diabetics, with, it is estimated, a probably equal number of folks who are diabetic without knowing it.

Rather recently scientists have become a bit more interested in another condition, which might loosely be called the opposite of diabetes—low blood sugar, otherwise known as hypoglycemia or hyperinsulinism. Ever so gradually some nutrition experts are coming to realize that the high sugar content of the average American diet may be having some rather serious effects on things other than tooth decay and obesity.

For, strangely enough—or perhaps not so strangely— the same good, high protein diet and frequent meals which protect the diabetic from disastrous variations in his blood sugar level, do exactly the same favor for those who suffer from low blood sugar. The object is to normalize the level of sugar in the blood at all times, before and after meals. To do this, a high protein diet is essential and frequent feedings are recommended.

We are also coming to realize that other things than food

have a considerable bearing on blood sugar levels: cigarettes, coffee, strong tea, soft drinks, emotional stress, violent exercise, and so forth. But the main interest still centers around what you eat and how often you eat it.

An excellent, easy-to-read book has been available for many years on this subject. Written by a man who suffered from low blood sugar and the doctor who cured him,* *Body, Mind and Sugar* is, according to a note on the jacket "your key to understanding alcoholism, neurosis, suicide, allergy, chronic fatigue, insanity . . . even murder." Not a word about overweight, but, as the foregoing quotes have shown you, perhaps overweight is the disease which will finally yield to the diet that controls low blood sugar or hypoglycemia.

In this book a full explanation is given of the way sugar —plain sugar—and to a lesser extent foods high in starches —upset the normal range of sugar levels in your blood so that you may, for a considerable part of each day, be trying to get along on too little sugar available in your blood to carry on the functions of blood sugar, one of the most important of which is to feed the brain and nerves.

Too little sugar in the blood! you exclaim. Well, then shouldn't I begin to eat more sugar rather than less? No. And herein lies one of the complexities of the body's use of sugar and starches which has not as yet interested many nutrition researchers many of whom continue to blame heredity and peculiarities of body structure for disasters that are obviously the result of years of abuse of one's body— and to a large extent the abuse of the body's blood sugar regulating mechanism.

An excellent chapter in *Body, Mind and Sugar* explains just how this mechanism works. The liver is involved and

* A. W. Pezet and E. M. Abrahamson, M.D. See bibliography.

many glands. The whole process of exactly what happens to sugar as it enters your digestive tract and proceeds along what the biochemists call "metabolic pathways" is diagrammed and outlined with great care. We need not go into the process here. Unless you want to read the book, you will just have to take our word for it that, when sugar and starch are presented to your digestive tract as a part of natural foods (and almost all foods contain some sugar and/or starch) considerable time is consumed in processing these foods, breaking them down into various secondary chemical forms. All the glandular and enzyme systems involved in this process automatically start their work, which, because of its very complex nature, results in sugar being released *ever so gradually* into the blood.

Where sugar and starch occur in food, they are accompanied by proteins, fats, vitamins, minerals, enzymes, and indigestible fibers, all of which slow down the process of assimilation and release of sugar to the blood and other places where it goes. These various food elements must be sorted out and each one sent to the processing depot where it is supposed to be.

During all the millions of years that living cells and tissues have been developing and all the millions of years that the digestive and assimilative systems of human beings have been developing, food was presented to human stomachs in the form of a complete, unfragmented package. Meat, seafood, eggs, fruits, berries, nuts and seeds, which appear to have been our original foods, are all mixtures of proteins, fats, starches, sugars, along with everything that naturally accompanies them. After we discovered how to grow cereal foods and vegetables, we still ate whole foods. Grains were pounded or ground, with nothing discarded except the inedible dry husks. Vegetables were eaten raw or cooked with

35

as much of their outer coatings and skins as could be digested by human systems.

Presumably glands and digestive juices, over these thousands of years, worked out the proper metabolic pathways for handling each new kind of food. Otherwise we would not have survived. But within the past several hundred years, due to man's vaunted ingenuity and technology, we developed ways to process foods into something they had never been before. We found out how to separate sugar completely from all the food elements that accompany it in growing things. It turned out to be a marvelous white substance which keeps indefinitely without refrigeration. And when it is added to foods in considerable amounts, it preserves them, too. And it tastes sweet!

Within the last 30 years or so, we have been using increasing amounts of this delightful white substance, until today "the average American" eats more than one hundred pounds of sugar a year. Since there are many millions of Americans who, because of special diets, eat almost no sugar, this figure is misleading. Those of us who do eat sugar manage to consume far more than 100 pounds a year of the sweet stuff. This in addition to the starches and sugars we get in fruits, vegetables and cereals.

There is no record anywhere of such a circumstance ever occurring before in the history of living things. Never have whole populations been subjected almost overnight to a biological experiment of such proportions.

The blood sugar regulating mechanism, purring along for millions of years with its tidy but complicated machinery for separating food elements and processing them ever so gradually, is suddenly presented with a completely new substance—pure sugar. This does not exist anywhere in nature. Nature has an apparent aversion to "pure" substances. Nature makes stones and rocks, mountains and seashores, trees and mosses—none of them "pure."

Now if such an obviously un-biological, un-natural substance as white sugar were mixed in small amounts with foods that naturally contain sugar, our blood sugar regulating mechanisms should have little difficulty in dealing with such foods. An apple made into applesauce and sweetened just a bit in the process is hardly more of a challenge to the blood sugar regulating mechanism than a very sweet whole apple.

And when human beings first had sugar, this is the way they used it. It was rare and expensive. It was considered a spice in the early days. And it was used sparingly as spices are used. Today, "pure" white sugar is just about the cheapest food you can buy. No wonder we eat so much of it. No wonder a whole mythology has grown up about this delicious food. "You must have sugar for energy." "You have to get a certain amount of sugar every day," and so on.

To get back to the blood sugar regulating mechanism. It is elaborate, delicately attuned, carefully balanced and intricately involved with almost every other part of the human body. Now picture such a delicate machine in a laboratory or a factory. Picture dumping into it, all of a sudden, a substance which has never been used in this particular machinery before. Any engineer will tell you that this would be madness. Yet this is, in essence, what we have done in the last 30 years or so in all the Western countries where sugar has become one of the cheapest foods you can buy.

Hypoglycemia, or low blood sugar, the condition talked about in *Body, Mind and Sugar,* appears to be one possible result. The elaborate mechanism which deals with regulating blood sugar is triggered violently by this sudden dumping of pure sugar. The level of blood sugar rises. This explains the "lift" you get from a candy bar or a soft drink. You feel better when your blood sugar level is high. Your nervousness tends to disappear, your hunger is appeased, your restlessness gone.

Fine, indeed, if things only stayed this way. But, because the sugar was released too rapidly into the blood, an inevitable fall ensues and the level of sugar in the blood is quite likely to plunge far below what you need to be comfortable. So in an hour, two hours or three, you are hungry again, nervous again, restless, inattentive. You need something to eat. Another candy bar, a sweet roll, a soft drink, a cup of coffee. Once again, after the lift and a swing upwards in blood sugar, you feel better.

In people whose blood sugar regulating mechanism has been damaged this kind of cycle may go on all day and far into the night. Dr. Abrahamson, in his book, relates low blood sugar levels to asthma attacks which may occur at night when the blood sugar has dropped far too low.

Other researchers have related low blood sugar to classic migraine headaches, which begin as soon as one awakes. This is the time when blood sugar levels may hit the lowest point. The headache is the symptom. In modern America it is almost a classic joke that lots of people can't really get started in the morning until they have a cup of coffee. According to Dr. Abrahamson, coffee acts much like sugar in triggering a swift rise in blood sugar levels which then may fall rapidly in a few hours.

What does all this have to do with losing weight? One of the things that happens when your blood sugar level sinks below what it should be is that you may feel hungry. Sugary foods seem to relieve this feeling better than any other kind so you eat more sugar, which produces the same effect and causes the same symptoms over and over. What is the answer?

The answer, according to Dr. Abrahamson and many other responsible scientists, is a diet high in protein and rather high in fat, taken in small meals at frequent intervals during the day so that you never get desperately hungry. The protein is satisfying and filling. As you begin to include more and more protein in your meals and between-meal snacks, your need for food slackens. Fat is digested very slowly. It leaves your stomach slowly. This is another reason why, with this kind of diet, you will avoid those aching hunger pangs, that feeling of light-headedness, that headache, that nervousness, that jittery feeling in your stomach that formerly caused you to seek out the coffee pot or open another bottle of soda.

The other excellent and sensible reason why this kind of diet reduces weight is that, as you eat more and more protein and fat you eat less and less of foods that give you nothing but calories—no vitamins, no minerals. And those are the foods that have been adding pounds, as well as practically guaranteeing that you will become an addict to such foods, needing more and more of them all the time.

Dr. Abrahamson relates almost unbelievable stories about the effect of the high-protein, low carbohydrate diet on alcoholics, on asthmatics, on allergics, on arthritics, on people with gout. He believes, he says, that crime statistics might be suddenly reduced if tests were done on potential criminals to search for low blood sugar curves. He tells of potential suicides treated with his diet who returned to complete good mental health. One of these was a woman who was "reducing" by eating only one meal a day and drinking coffee all day long to keep going. Says Dr. Abrahamson,

"Such a diet almost guarantees hyperinsulism," or low blood sugar.

So perhaps many of the desperate overweight folks who are trying today to lose weight by skipping meals and drinking coffee or soft drinks all day are in fact doing themselves just about the worst damage they could do, for they are almost guaranteeing such an insult to their blood sugar regulating mechanism that they may pay for it in much worse disorders in the future.

The diet Dr. Abrahamson prescribes for his low blood sugar patients is very simple and easy to follow. It specifies only that you omit sugar and starchy foods and that you eat frequently during the day. It goes like this:

When you get up in the morning have a medium orange, a half grapefruit or four ounces of citrus or tomato juice.

At breakfast, eat fruit or four ounces of juice, one egg with or without two slices of ham or bacon. One slice of bread or toast with plenty of butter. Beverage. No coffee. Two hours after breakfast, have four ounces of citrus juice or tomato juice.

For lunch have meat, fish, cheese or eggs plus a salad with plenty of salad dressing, plus the allowable vegetables if you want them, ONLY ONE slice of bread with plenty of butter. Dessert and beverage. See below for the desserts and drinks that are permitted.

Three hours after lunch, have 8 ounces of milk.

One hour before dinner, have four ounces of citrus or tomato juice.

For dinner, have soup, if you wish. It must not, of course, contain any of the forbidden vegetables or starches. And a liberal portion of meat, fish, or poultry plus the permitted vegetables, ONLY ONE slice of bread if desired, dessert and beverage.

Two to three hours after dinner have 8 ounces of milk.

Every two hours until bedtime, have four ounces of milk or a small handful of nuts.

Within the framework of this method of spacing meals and snacks, here is a list of forbidden foods, along with those of which you are encouraged to eat as much as you want:

Allowable vegetables: asparagus, avocado, beets, broccoli, brussels sprouts, cabbage, cauliflower, carrots, celery, corn, cucumbers, eggplant, lima beans, onions, peas, radishes, sauerkraut, squash, string beans, tomatoes, turnips.

Allowable fruits: apples, apricots, berries, grapefruit, melons, oranges, peaches, pears, pineapple, tangerines.

These may be cooked or raw, with or without cream, but *without any sugar. Canned fruits must be water-packed, not in syrup.*

Lettuce and other salad greens, mushrooms and nuts may be eaten as freely as desired.

Fruit juice may be any *unsweetened* juice, except grape juice or prune juice.

Beverages: weak tea (made with a tea ball, not brewed), decaffeinated coffee, coffee substitutes. Any of these may be sweetened with artificial sweeteners.

Desserts: fruit, unsweetened gelatin, junket made from tablets, not mix.

Alcoholic and soft drinks: Club soda, dry ginger ale, whiskies or other distilled liquors.

These foods must be avoided absolutely: sugar, candy and all other sweets, such as cake, pie, pastries, sweet cus-

tards, puddings and ice cream. This of course includes such doubtful items as chewing gum, which contains sugar.

You must also avoid caffeine in any form such as strong brewed tea, coffee or soft drinks that contain it.

You must avoid potatoes, rice, grapes, raisins, figs, dates and bananas.

You must avoid spaghetti, macaroni and noodles. We would add to this every other kind of food made with flour such as pizza, etc. You must avoid wines, cordials and beer.

Dr. Abrahamson is making no effort here to prescribe a reducing diet. To take off weight, in addition to regulating blood sugar levels, it would seem wise, wouldn't it, to substitute foods with a bit less carbohydrate for some that he allows. For instance, tomato juice contains about one-third the carbohydrate of orange, grapefruit or apple juice. It would seem sensible to substitute it for the other juices.

Sorting out the vegetables, you find that all the allowed ones are reasonably low in carbohydrate except for corn, lima beans and peas. It would be a good idea for the dieter to skip these. Although Dr. Abrahamson does not mention them, all the wonderful crisp, crunchy salad vegetables are allowed in any quantity.

Of the fruits, it would seem sensible, wouldn't it, to use only those which we know are lowest in carbohydrates. This would be the melon family chiefly.

Dr. Abrahamson allows his patients to have one slice of bread or toast at every meal. For the reducer, surely one-half slice a meal, or no bread at all would be preferable. You'll be amazed at how easy it is to do without bread, once you start, since you are allowed to eat all you want of other filling foods like meat, fish, poultry and so forth. Dr. Abrahamson allows crackers and cheese for dessert. The

42

reducer would certainly skip the crackers. You can easily eat cheese quite alone—as much as you want. You can perch a slice of it on a slice of pepper, celery, avocado, cucumber. You can spread soft cheese like cottage cheese on almost any vegetable.

Dr. John W. Tintera of Yonkers, New York, worked with alcoholics for more than twenty years. In the many articles he wrote on this disease, he stated that the crux of the alcoholic's problem is low blood sugar. Many alcoholics refer to their early childhood liking for candy and other sweets. They confess to going on binges of sweets-eating. Depression and fatigue were temporarily cured that way, they found. The craving for sweets is a manifestation of low blood sugar, says Dr. Tintera. Alcoholics have found that alcohol can produce the same relaxing effect as sugar.

All the alcoholics he has examined were suffering from low blood sugar. He points out again and again in his writings that the important thing in dealing with low blood sugar is not the point *from* which the blood sugar level falls, or the point *to* which it falls, *but rather the suddenness of the fall*. This is the reason for the discomfort, the craving for sugar or alcohol and all the other symptoms. The high-protein, moderate-fat diet, in which the quickly absorbed starches and sweets (that is, the refined ones, remember!) are eliminated entirely, tends to alleviate these sudden plunges from one level to another. Protein is assimilated slowly by the body. Fat is assimilated slowly.

You can get more information about Dr. Tintera's treatment for alcoholism by writing to: Adrenal Metabolic Research Society of the Hypoglycemia Foundation, Inc., P. O. Box 98, Fleetwood, Mount Vernon, New York, 10552.

Dr. Tintera gives this diet list:

Foods Allowed:

All meats, fowl, fish and shellfish
Dairy products (eggs, milk, butter and cheese)
All vegetables and fruits not mentioned below
Salted nuts (excellent between meals)
Peanut butter, oat and jerusalem artichoke bread
Gelatin with whipped cream
Sanka, weak tea and sugar-free soft drinks
Soybeans and soybean products
Oatmeal
Certain high-protein macaroni and spaghetti

Foods to avoid:

Potatoes, corn, macaroni, spaghetti, rice, cereals
Pie, cake, pastries, sugar, candies
Dates, raisins and other dried fruits
Cola and other sweet soft drinks
Coffee and strong tea
Alcohol in all forms

The foods allowed were chosen for their high protein content. Soybeans and peanuts, for instance, are also high in carbohydrate. But Dr. Tintera apparently feels that their protein content will assure the dieter that the carbohydrate is released ever so gradually during the process of digestion, so that it cannot damage the delicate balance of the blood sugar regulating mechanism.

Read the diet carefully. It looks very much like the other diets described in this book, doesn't it? Nothing is said about how much of any food one should eat, since, we are sure, Dr. Tintera has found that after a few weeks on the diet no one has any wish to overeat. The kinds of foods he recommends have their own built-in guarantee against eating too much.

What does a diet for curing alcoholics have to do with reducers? Note the craving for sweets so often reported by alcoholics. Sound familiar? Do you know anybody who tells you "I just can't get through the afternoon without a candy bar"? "I must have my prune danish at ten every morning or I can't make it till lunch time"? This is the same craving for sweets which, in the alcoholic, develops into alcoholism. It is the direct result of a chronic low blood sugar condition. It can be overcome by the same diet that cures the alcoholic.

If the low carbohydrate, high-protein diet is a powerful enough regulator of body mechanisms to control completely the alcoholic's craving for alcohol, doesn't it seem much more than likely that it can control an unbalanced craving for sugar and starch?

Benjamin P. Sandler of the Departments of Medicine and Pathology, Veterans Administration Hospital, Oteen, North Carolina, recently treated a patient with subacute bacterial endocarditis with a high-protein, low-carbohydrate diet, while he was giving him antibiotics, and reports that the patient's temperature was normal within 24 hours and his blood showed "early and persistent" decrease in bacteria. Dr. Sandler believes that the diet had a great deal to do with the patient's rapid recovery from the fever.

This is not surprising, for Dr. Sandler has been advocating this diet for many years. In 1940 he published a paper in *The Review of Gastroenterology* on controlling the pain of ulcers with a low carbohydrate diet. In 1941 he published a paper on chronic abdominal pain due to hypoglycemia, or low blood sugar and a paper on the low carbohydrate diet in controlling angina pectoris, the pain of a certain heart condition. In 1942 and 1950 he published papers on the treatment of tuberculosis with a low carbohydrate diet. In 1951 he published a book, *Diet Prevents Polio*—the low carbohydrate diet, that is. This book tells the story of a local polio epidemic which was stopped in its tracks within a few days after Dr. Sandler went on the local radio with recommendations for eliminating high-carbohydrate foods from the children's meals.

In 1958 he published a book, *How To Prevent Heart Attacks*. This is not a book on reducing, although Dr. Sandler does say that patients of his who eat his suggested diet lose weight if they are overweight, and gain weight if they are too thin. One could hardly ask for a better recommendation for a diet.

He tells us in this book that since 1937 he has performed hundreds of tests on patients to search for low blood sugar tendencies. *He says he has found evidence of low blood sugar levels in more than half of them.* He has found, too, that a diet aimed to correct the low blood sugar did away with or greatly alleviated many symptoms not only in patients whose blood sugar levels were low, but in those who appeared to have normal levels. "I have concluded," he says, "that any human can experience low blood sugar as long as he or she consumes sugar and starch."

He says that many healthy people have symptoms of low blood sugar without realizing it. At about eleven in the morning and around four in the afternoon they have a "letdown." They may get a slight headache, feel fatigued, depressed, light-headed or hungry. They want something sweet. After a snack of candy or cake, pie, soft drinks or coffee, there is a rapid rise in the blood sugar and the symptoms are relieved.

"I regard as artificial the rapid rise in blood sugar level produced by eating foods containing sugar," says Dr. Sandler. "The sugar is an artificial stimulant; and in some people the desire for sweets amounts to a craving, and the demand for something sweet during this craving amounts to an addiction. I regard this craving for sweets as abnormal. . . . The low blood sugar that comes on around 11 a.m. is due to eating sugar or starch at breakfast, and the low blood sugar at 4 p.m. is due to eating sugar and starch at the noon meal. On a high-protein, low-carbohydrate diet the fall in blood sugar at 11 a.m. and 4 p.m. does not occur and so there is no physical let-down and no need for a pick-up. Cigarette smoking can also serve as a pick-up because nicotine can cause an immediate rise in blood sugar level by stimulating the adrenal-sympathetic system, the rise occuring at the expense of liver glycogen."

Dr. Sandler goes on to say, "The desire for a cigarette actually coincides with a fall in blood sugar and the feeling of satisfaction that comes with a smoke is due to a rise in blood sugar. Denicotinized cigarettes do not satisfy because they do not cause a rise in blood sugar." Coffee, tea, cocoa not only cause a rise in blood sugar by reason of the added sugar, but also because they contain caffeine or related chemical compounds that stimulate the adrenal-sympathetic system and thus cause a rise in blood sugar at the expense of liver glycogen.

Dr. Sandler believes that the low-carbohydrate diet is as beneficial to the person with low blood sugar as to the person who is diabetic and hence has blood sugar levels that are generally too high. In both cases, it regulates the levels so that wide fluctuations are eliminated. In this way, he says, the heart is assured of adequate delivery of sugar at all times and is not exposed to sudden unexpected lowering of the blood sugar.

It is Dr. Sandler's belief that this sudden lessening of the supply of sugar to the heart is the leading cause of heart attacks in this country. He produces some extremely convincing case histories to justify this claim. In case after case, symptoms of pending heart attacks are relieved by following the recommended diet. They return when the diet is broken and a few teaspoons of sugar or a few slices of bread are added at every meal. His chapter on smoking should be required reading for every smoker. It not only gives a graphic picture of what happens to you when you smoke—both after meals and "on an empty stomach"—but it recommends the best possible way to give up smoking. Regulate your blood sugar levels with a low-carbohydrate diet and you will find that the addictive craving for cigarettes disappears. It's just that simple.

Dr. Sandler also takes up the effects of unpleasant, anxious or psychological stresses on blood sugar levels. Bad news may send the levels way down. Sudden emergencies or shocks, unaccustomed heavy work (snow shovelling comes to mind) may deplete the blood of necessary sugar. While we may feel a need for getting through such a crisis by eating something sweet or drinking coffee, the only sensible food to take instead is protein food which will stabilize the blood sugar levels and hence protect us to some extent from the effects of the stress.

How long should one stay on the diet Dr. Sandler recommends? Why not for good? Why go back to the old sugary days with all kinds of unpleasant symptoms? But don't you "need" sugar for energy? Of course you do, and the best way to get that sugar to the proper place—the brain, the heart, the liver—at the proper time is to eat foods which will release the sugar ever so gradually into the blood, not dump it precipitously at the wrong time and in the wrong place.

Dr. Sandler says, "I have thus found that a diet completely

free of sugar and starch and consisting of proteins, fats and nonstarchy vegetables, may be adhered to for years with beneficial effects and absolutely without harmful effects. There is no supporting evidence to indicate that sugar and starch are necessary for health or for energy purposes. The human is a carnivore and can thrive on protein and fat alone, if necessary." Does that sound familiar?

One last and very significant note on the subject of heart disease. This is not the subject of this book, but it is, it *has* to be, a subject of more than passing interest to every American, for at present heart attacks claim more lives than any other disorder. Many of these people are young, apparently healthy, full of hopes and dreams. The heart attack changes all that.

In 1956, in the *American Journal of the Medical Sciences*, an article appeared on coronary heart disease (the condition that brings on heart attacks) written by three men, one of whom is a leading heart specialist, Dr. Paul Dudley White. Another author is Dr. Fredrick Stare, head of Harvard University's department of nutrition. These gentlemen stated, "To realize that the first cause of death in the United States is a disease little known 50 years ago comes as something of a surprise to physicians and public alike. . . . No disease has ever come so quickly from obscurity to the place coronary heart disease now occupies, to maintain itself there with a permanence presumably to endure in this country for years to come."

They are surprised, you see, that this disorder appears to have come stalking out of nowhere within the past 50 years. The question of what causes it is at present occupying some of the best scientific minds in the country. Maybe we sit too much, they speculate. We eat the wrong kind of fat. We smoke too much. We are exposed to too much stress. Air pollution may be doing it. Or the minerals in our water supply.

Only in very recent years have a number of capable and courageous researchers begun to present evidence implicating the enormous increase in the sugar and starch in our diets as the cause of heart attacks. *This increase has occurred only within the past 50 years or so.* Why not face it and conduct some far-reaching investigations to discover what the results may be?

Until this is done, through some national project where diets will be closely supervised, why not take advantage of what we now know, through the work of the medical men referred to in this book? While you are losing weight, why not perhaps put off the day you can expect that heart attack?

Dr. Sandler's diet, which puts his heart patients back on the road to health, which takes off weight from fatties and puts it back on the beanpoles, is a very simple diet to follow.

All animal foods may be eaten in unlimited quantity. That's right—unlimited quantity. Any meats, seafood or poultry, fresh, canned, smoked, dried. Eggs can be eaten in unlimited quantity. All dairy products may be eaten in unlimited quantity. Fresh fruits are allowed but only one portion should be eaten at a meal, since they contain considerable sugar. Fruit juices, canned fruits, dried fruits, preserved fruits are forbidden. Fruits may be stewed without sugar. Apples may be baked without sugar. Tomato juice can be taken freely since it contains no natural sugar.

He then lists carbohydrate foods which may be eaten in unlimited quantity: artichokes, asparagus, avocados, bamboo shoots, string beans and wax beans, soy beans, red beans, broccoli, brussels sprouts, cabbage, cauliflower, celery, chard, collards, cucumbers, eggplant, endive, greens of any kind, kale, kohlrabi, leeks, lettuce, mushrooms, okra, onions, parsley, parsnips, peas (fresh), peppers, pumpkins, radishes, rhubarb, rutabaga, sorrel, spinach, squash (summer) tomatoes, turnips, watercress, pickles, horseradish, mustard, vinegar, olives, capers, mayonnaise.

These foods, high in carbohydrate should be eaten *in reduced quantity:* dried beans (baked, for instance), lima beans, tapioca, macaroni, rolls, crackers, corn, dried split peas, potatoes (white or sweet) yams, lentils, rice, spaghetti, vermicelli, noodles, all breads, buns, biscuits and cereals.

The following foods should be entirely avoided: sugar, soft drinks, ice cream, ices, sherbets, cakes, candies, cookies, wafers, pastries, pies, fruit juices, canned and preserved fruits, jams, jellies, marmalades, puddings, custards, syrups.

Coffee, tea and cocoa, lemonade and so forth may be sweetened with artificial sweeteners. "Diabetic foods and desserts" may be eaten. Nuts may be eaten in unlimited quantity except for peanuts, cashews and chestnuts which may be eaten sparingly.

For meals, Dr. Sandler suggests this for breakfast: fresh fruit or tomato juice, two or more eggs, if desired, plus ham, bacon, fish, cheese or other meat, no more than one slice of bread with butter. Beverage without sugar. Lunch consists of tomato juice or soup with no starchy fillers, as much as you wish of meat, fish or poultry and any of the permitted vegetables, with no more than one slice of bread and butter, one piece of fresh fruit and beverage. Dinner is the same, with added salad and nuts and cheese permitted along with your piece of fresh fruit. Isn't it, in essence, the same diet endorsed in this book?

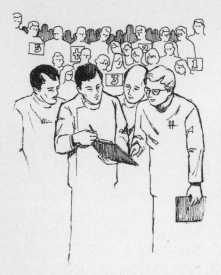

CHAPTER SIX

A VERY CRUDE EXPERIMENT —THE ONLY DIFFERENCE WAS SUGAR

W HAT THEY DESCRIBE as "a very crude experiment" was performed in 1967 by two doctors and two dentists at the University of Alabama Medical Center and reported in the *Alabama Journal of Medical Sciences,* July, 1967. Dr. E. Cheraskin and three associates conducted an experiment in weight loss or gain, using 121 dental students as subjects.

They weighed each one on Monday, then divided them into five groups. The first group was given 50 grams of sucrose in solution twice daily under supervision, to be sure that it was taken. Fifty grams of sucrose is about one-fourth cup of sugar, plain white sugar. The second group received no special addition to their diet. The third group had, every day, 75 grams of glucose (another kind of sugar) in a drink. The fourth group received three times daily a drink containing no calories whatsoever but which looked exactly like the drink given to group 3. The fifth group of students were told to eliminate from their meals all foods that contained refined carbohydrates. This means everything that has white sugar, white flour or processed cereals in it. All desserts, except fruit, all pasta, noodles, bread, muffins, biscuits, doughnuts, and so forth, and all cereals. At the end of the week, all students were once again weighed by someone who had no knowledge of which students had been eating what kind of diets during the week.

In the space of one week, half of the students who were getting the sugar gained weight. The average weight gain was one-half pound. In the third group more than half of the students gained weight—eight-tenths of a pound on the average. Of the students who eliminated all refined carbo-hydrates from their meals, 63 per cent lost weight—an average of 1.2 pounds. IN ONE WEEK!

The authors tell us what this would mean in the course of a month. The students adding just one-fourth cup of plain sugar to their meals could be expected to gain two pounds in a month. By the end of the year this would be about 24 pounds. *Note, please, that they made no other change at all in their eating habits.* They ate the same amount of meat, eggs, milk, potatoes and everything else—but they added just ¼ cup of white sugar.

What would you have to eat to add one-fourth cup of sugar in the course of one day's meals? One-fourth cup is 12 teaspoons. A soft drink may contain five teaspoons. A piece of apple pie may contain 12. A doughnut contains five teaspoons. So adding two soft drinks a day, a piece of pie or two doughnuts in addition to your regular diet could be expected to make you about 24 pounds heavier within the year.

By skipping all refined carbohydrates *and making no other change in your diet,* you might be expected to lose

53

something like 4.8 pounds a month, or *more than 57 pounds in the course of a year!* Note, please, that no one counted calories in this experiment. No one even followed the students around to make sure that they kept strictly to the letter of the law in abjuring refined carbohydrates. Note that no one was asked to give up such foods as potatoes, beans, carrots, or any kind of fruit. So the reduction was not even achieved by cutting down on *all* high-carbohydrate foods. Just the refined carbohydrates, by which is meant those foods which have been drastically changed and concentrated in the processing. White flour is the result of milling which removes most of the germ of the wheat. The germ contains most of the protein, the vitamins, minerals and unsaturated fats. The flour that is left has thus been concentrated into being mostly carbohydrate, with little else that accompanies it in the natural grain.

White sugar is arrived at by removing just about *everything* that occurs in the sugarcane or sugar beet, except the carbohydrate. Such a food as this never occurs in nature. According to many authorities whom we have quoted in this book, the tongue, the appestat, the blood sugar mechanism of the human being do not know how to deal with this kind of so-called food, because, over the years of evolution, no such food has ever been available before.

All that Dr. Cheraskin and his colleagues were trying to find out was whether the refined carbohydrates make you fat. And leaving the refined carbohydrates out of your meals makes you thin. Admittedly the evidence of a one-week experiment, when nobody was followed around to see what they actually ate, is "a crude experiment." On the other hand, if this much average weight can be lost or gained in the course of only a week, doesn't this show that more exact experiments where every mouthful is measured and weighed and large groups of people are followed for months or years might prove even more conclusively that the heart of the trouble is indeed the refined carbohydrates?

So long as you continue to try to reduce by cutting calories, there is no way to test this theory of the Alabama researchers. For if you are going to take a considerable part or even a small part of your calories in refined carbohydrate form, your body will continue to be unable to deal with these foods, you will continue to suffer hunger pangs and you're bound to give up on the whole project. One piece of candy or one sticky bun may not necessarily add so many calories to your day's total that they would cause a weight gain. But the upheaval in your blood sugar mechanism that follows such foods may do all the damage, for you're faint, you're tired, you're unable to work. By golly, you just have to have another bite of something sweet to keep going! So you do.

Dr. Cheraskin and his friends at Alabama University have been doing a lot of investigating of the refined carbohydrates and reporting their findings regularly. In one experiment (*Journal of the Medical Association of the State of Alabama,* September, 1965) they reported that analysis of blood sugar levels and blood pressure showed that both these vital body processes fluctuate during the day and that the patterns of fluctuation depend on the intake of refined carbohydrate foods. *When sugar and white flour foods are reduced, fluctuations in blood sugar and blood pressure diminish.* In other words, by removing just these two categories of foods from meals, they can achieve "homeostasis" —that healthful condition when everything is in balance and purring along the way it's supposed to.

In the 1965 *Journal of Oral Therapeutics,* they reported on the effect on mouth and gum health of drinks containing sugar. Seventy-six dental students participated. Forty of these were told to eat a high-protein diet with consumption of refined carbohydrate foods cut to a minimum. Twenty-two students were told to eat their usual diet but to add drinks containing ¼ cup of sugar twice daily. A third group were told to eat as they usually did and add nothing to their diets. At the end of only four days the dentist who examined their gums at the beginning of the experiment examined them again without knowing which of the students had been eating which diet. He found that the students who took the sugar drink had worse gum conditions, those who ate the high protein diet had better conditions. *In the space of only four days!* Once again, the authors apologize for the roughness of the experiment. But there is no denying what it showed. In similar experiments, the mobility of teeth was studied—that is, how firmly attached they were to the gums. Here again, the students who took the sugary drinks had a considerable increase in tooth mobility—loose teeth, that is.

Specialists in diabetes are alarmed when they study the patterns of blood sugar levels in the older people in our country. As age goes up, the blood sugar levels appear to go up, too, seeming to indicate that older folks are more and more tending toward diabetic states with all the attendant perils in the way of heart and artery trouble, blindness, infections, and so on. Dr. Cheraskin's group in the April, 1966 issue of the *Alabama Journal of Medical Science,* reports on almost 9000 citizens tested for blood sugar levels in a Diabetes Detection Drive.

The immediate observation in the study, say the authors, is that blood sugar levels tend to rise with advancing age. But, they go on, the figures also show that, as we grow older, we also tend to show more *low* blood sugar figures than those who are in younger age groups. If we believe that

56

higher blood sugar readings are not just a natural part of aging, they argue, then we must believe that older folks are relatively often subject to this disorder. If one grants that diabetic (that is, high) blood sugar levels are part of aging and most of us can expect to develop them, then we have to admit, as well, that low blood sugar levels are also comparatively frequent among older folks.

Dr. Cheraskin's group, being scientists, do not step out of their strictly scientific roles to hazard any guesses as to why these conditions might be. But doesn't it seem possible that the kind of food these folks have been eating over the years may have a great deal to do with these two opposite conditions, both of them troublesome in the extreme? Diabetes and diabetic complications are responsible for many deaths. We do not as yet know the full extent of disorders caused by *low* blood sugar.

The Alabama group of researchers, in 1967, investigated a group of patients at an Alabama hospital suffering from cancer. They carefully matched them against another group of completely healthy dental students. Then they tested the blood sugar levels of both groups. Twice as many of the cancer patients had elevated blood sugar levels. And the average levels of blood sugar at every point along the way were higher in the group of people suffering from cancer.

Diabetes and its opposite, low blood sugar, are directly related to the body's use of carbohydrates. Too high or too low levels of blood sugar indicate that the body cannot deal successfully with carbohydrate foods. An ever-increasing number of Americans are showing these tendencies. There are already millions of us who are diabetics and more millions who are probable diabetics or pre-diabetics.

In another experiment, Dr. Cheraskin and his colleagues interviewed a group of 74 dentists and their wives, asking questions about their diets and their heart and artery complaints. The diet questions pinpointed how much each person eats of non-refined foods high in carbohydrate—foods like potatoes, beans, nuts; and how much each person eats of highly refined foods like sugar, white bakery products, desserts; how much vegetable protein and how much animal protein. Then each individual was asked 13 questions which are considered to be indicative of the condition of one's heart and arteries, such questions as "has a doctor ever said your blood pressure is too high?" and so on.

They found that the folks who ate the most of the refined carbohydrates and the least protein and natural carbohydrate-high foods had the most cardiovascular complaints. Again, this was a small sample of people, but the survey was professionally and carefully done, and reported in the *Journal of Oral Medicine* for January, 1968. What might be revealed by a survey among several thousand people?

The close relation between the eating of sugar, especially refined white sugar, and other refined carbohydrates and many assorted disorders, from gum troubles to diabetes and possibly cancer, is clearly shown in Dr. Cheraskin's work. Wouldn't it be a fairly good idea to cut out as much sugar and refined carbohydrates from your meals as you can, whether you are overweight or not?

CHAPTER SEVEN

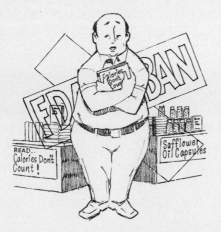

CALORIES DO COUNT OR ONE FOOT IS A LOT DIFFERENT THAN TEN FEET

ON JULY 7, 1962 an astonishing report appeared on the front page of the *New York Times*. George Larrick, Commissioner of the Food and Drug Administration, announced that the best-selling book, *Calories Don't Count,* by Herman Taller, M.D. was deliberately created and used to promote sales of "worthless safflower oil capsules." 280 cases of safflower oil capsules had been seized, he said, along with copies of the book.

Said Mr. Larrick, "The freedom to publish health books is a constitutional guarantee. But, the courts held that books used to promote the commercialization of drugs become labeling under the Food, Drug and Cosmetic Act. False statements in the book misbrand the drugs."

The "drugs" in this case, for those of you who are not used to FDA nomenclature, are the safflower oil capsules which were seized. Since they had been displayed in some

59

stores, along with the book, *Calories Don't Count,* they were called drugs by the FDA and the book was called "labeling" of these drugs. The labeling of drugs must be exact, the FDA states, and hence an exact dosage of safflower oil had to be prescribed by Dr. Taller, author of the book. And furthermore, Dr. Taller had to have "scientific evidence" that this "drug" would do what he said it would do—that is, reduce weight.

This, in essence, is what the whole furor over *Calories Don't Count* comes down to. Later in the *Times* article Mr. Larrick announced that Dr. Taller had not written the book at all, but that it was prepared by "laymen" and one of its main purposes was to "promote the sale of a commercial product in which Dr. Taller had a financial interest."

Traditionally, the Food and Drug Administration works in a fearful and wonderful way its duties to perform. But *l'affaire Taller* sets a number of records, even for the FDA. Dr. Taller was later arrested, brought to trial and sentenced. The book, which no government bureau could proscribe, due to the first amendment, is still available, but is not being widely advertised.

Suffice it to say that the controversy which raged around *Calories Don't Count* must have set the health of the American people back by some ten or fifteen years, because what went on was, by the most charitable of definitions, sheer idiocy.

The financial dealings of Dr. Taller and the people who sold safflower oil are certainly of little concern to the millions of hopelessly overweight Americans and are, properly, not a fit subject for comment by someone interested only in nutrition and a wholesome and harmless way of reducing.

The content of Dr. Taller's book and what became of it *is* of interest. The book hit the top of the best seller list with the impact of a ten-ton truck and stayed there for months. Backed up by generous advertising on the part of the publisher, it was making headlines. No one will ever know, of course, how many people actually followed the diet suggested in the pages of this book, along with suggestions on things other than diet, and lost weight, thereby. Nor will anyone ever know how many people did *not* lose weight after following Dr. Taller's suggestions.

Columnists talked about it. Overweight actors and writers recommended it. People by the millions apparently took it quite seriously and gave it a whirl. Dr. Taller was a medical man, a gynecologist. The idea of his diet was, simply, to cut carbohydrates to the bare minimum and eat as much fat and protein as you wanted. The book also made a number of other restrictions which were generally lost sight of by reviewers and attackers in the pitched battles which ensued on editorial pages and in the columns of medical journals. Dr. Taller recommended cutting down on salt. He also recommended walking or some other quite vigorous exercise *for an hour every day*. He thought you should confine yourself to three meals a day.

The recommendation that you eat as much fat as you wish ran headlong into the frenzied controversy that was at that time taking place concerning the role of animal fat in the diet. One school of scientific thought had come to believe that animal fat is harming us. Cholesterol was the word they used. It should be outlawed or almost outlawed, they said. Another school of thought said that, well, we'd better cut down a little on animal fat because it is mainly "saturated," but at the same time we'd better add some "unsaturated" fats to balance the "saturated" kind. Just coming into sight over the top of the next ridge of scientific controversy was a group of researchers who were preparing to announce *that probably too much sugar, not fat at all,* is causing most of our circulatory ills.

Caught squarely in the middle were the American Medical Association, the American Heart Society and the National Academy of Sciences—three arbiters whose scientific opinions generally set the scientific tone for the nation. They were at odds. The AMA and the Heart people couldn't agree. The NAS didn't make up its collective mind until much later—1966 in fact, when they published an official booklet—*Dietary Fat and Human Health.*

Most of the American people hadn't a notion of what was going on and cared less. Generally speaking, some people probably began to pour a little more salad oil in their skillets in place of butter or lard. The dairy industry wrung its hands and protested to its congressmen. The salad oil industry sent smugly worded ads to the medical journals not quite claiming that eating lots of salad oil will save you from heart attacks, but almost claiming that. University professors who are supported by financial grants from the dairy industry attacked the theory that animal fats could do you in. Those professors supported by financial grants from people who make salad oil fought back.

Dr. Taller apparently decided to say in his book that much of the fat permissible on his recommended diet should probably be "unsaturated." Because safflower oil is highest in linoleic acid, which at the time seemed to be most effective in reducing levels of cholesterol in the blood, he recommended taking a certain amount of safflower oil every day. You could pour this over salad, use it for frying or braising, or drink it from a glass. The way in which you ingested it was not important to the plot.

Presumably many people who might be interested in the CDC diet wouldn't be able to control the fat content of their

62

diets quite this closely. Let's say they traveled and ate in a different restaurant every day. Or whoever did the cooking at home just couldn't be bothered to fiddle around with a certain kind of oil and spoil all her best recipes. So, said Dr. Taller, if you want to take safflower oil in capsules, that's all right, too.

This was the point at which the hanky-panky began. Some people apparently came to believe that all you had to do to reduce on the CDC diet was to eat whatever you wanted and drink some safflower oil, because safflower oil was a "miracle food." *Nothing could be farther from the content of Dr. Taller's book.*

The confusion—most of it quite purposeful confusion— around what Dr. Taller's book said and what it did not say is probably best illustrated by an editorial in the *Journal of the American Medical Association* which stated that "he recommended a diet for obese persons consisting principally of unsaturated fats."

There is still no indication that anyone on the staff of the *JAMA* has ever read the book or has any idea of what the recommended diet is. There is very little evidence that most of the people who reviewed the book in dietetic and medical journals had read it or understood what the diet really was. There is a lot of evidence that every effort was made by almost everyone concerned in the controversy to confuse the American public into believing that Dr. Taller—that fraud, that deceiver, that unscientific opportunist—had really said in the book that you could reduce *by simply eating anything you want, plus a lot of salad oil!* Nothing could be farther from the truth.

The *Journal of the American Medical Association* (July 21, 1962) printed a story, describing the seizures that were made by the FDA of the books and safflower capsules. They

63

quoted Mr. Larrick's statements at length, reporting that Taller's county medical society was urging action against him. In addition they printed an extraordinary interview with a deputy director of the FDA in which the following came to light. In a large drugstore where *Calories Don't Count* might be displayed in the book section and some safflower oil capsules displayed in the drug section, could the books then be seized? Mr. Milstead of the FDA said (yes, he really said this) that it depends on how far away the book is from the capsules. "One foot is a lot different than 10 feet," he said.

He went on to say (this is Mr. Milstead, as reported in the *Journal of the American Medical Association*) that if a customer asks a book section clerk whether the store sells the capsules and the clerk directs him to the drug section then that constitutes an argument for regarding the book as labeling. So the book and the capsules could be seized.

There is more. Mr. Milstead went on to say that "if a druggist has in his physical possession an advertising mat for a product, that would be evidence for 'labeling,' even if he kept the mat in his closet and didn't show it to anybody." His next statement is a bit ambiguous. He said that the FDA had already seized safflower oil mayonnaise and salad dressing, "dietetic crackers" (whatever that means) and safflower margarine and would proceed against "any other safflower, gluten or polyunsaturated fat products" wherever they were sold in association with the book. That means, according to what Mr. Milstead said above, if they were within, would you opine, ten feet of the book, or nine feet?

As we said earlier, the ways of the FDA are fearful and wonderful, and the infectious nature of their hates becomes apparent when one studies closely some of the articles which followed their original denunciation of Taller's book.

In the *JAMA* it was reviewed by the AMA expert on

nutrition, Dr. Philip L. White, a Doctor of Science. He said that Dr. Taller had written a book "that will rank high on the list representing nutrition nonsense and food quackery." He went on to quote Dr. John Yudkin of London University as saying that people on "such diets" consume fewer total calories than they had been accustomed to consume.

"In fact," says he, "several subjects consumed less fat on the high-fat diet. All patients lost weight, as would be expected on a reduced calorie intake. This study and others suggest that the high-fat diet of Taller, probably because of its appetite satisfaction, induces the individual to consume fewer calories than would be the case on a diet containing the usual level of carbohydrate."

This is precisely the whole theme of Dr. Taller's book. In fact he states specifically that the body has a built-in protection against eating too much fat. Too much fat nauseates you. So, if you are eating fat for calories instead of carbohydrate, you can't possibly eat too many calories. Hence, the catchy title *Calories Don't Count*.

Dr. White, alas, goes on to say, "The title of the book is most unfortunate and misleading. Calories do count." This brings us to the crux of the matter. What everybody objected to was the title. And apparently most people who reviewed the book anywhere or who objected to its contents seldom read very far beyond the title. The *JAMA* which gloated over Dr. Taller's downfall, printed a cartoon from the *New Yorker* in which CDC was displayed in a window surrounded by pastries, cakes and cookies—as if this was the kind of diet Dr. Taller recommended!

The diet recommended in *Calories Don't Count* is simply this: You are permitted, nay, encouraged, to eat

all meats (trim off visible fat)
all forms of seafood, with the natural oils and fats

all kinds of cheese
only those vegetables that contain no more than 5 per
    cent carbohydrate. A list of 29 vegetables is given,
    all low in carbohydrate
eggs, fried in margarine or unsaturated oils
gluten bread (low in carbohydrate)
fruit containing less than 5 per cent carbohydrate
nuts in the shell
coffee, tea, diet soft drinks or milk (one cup daily)

You may not eat anything else. At lunch you must eat at least 6 to 8 ounces of meat, poultry, fish or seafood. At dinner you must eat at least ten to twelve ounces. And you must eat a specified amount of additional fat in the form of salad oil and margarine.

You must eat three meals a day and you must drink considerable amounts of water—at least three glasses between one meal and the next, says Dr. Taller. Fish or shellfish are to be eaten at least once a day, because they are rich in the unsaturated fats.

This is the diet that brought down on itself all the fury of the Food and Drug Administration and the "establishment" authorities on nutrition. There is no way of telling how much of this fury may have been caused by the fact that the CDC diet forbids absolutely all those foods on which the food industry makes its greatest profits. There is no way of knowing how much money the sugar industry and the flour industry, the baking industry, the soft drink and candy people lost during the days when *Calories Don't Count* topped the best seller list month after month.

It seems clear that the general public was left with the distinct impression that the diet was a fraud, that no one could possibly lose weight by following it and that it might, in fact, be quite dangerous. Of course there is not a shred of scientific evidence that any of these things is true. But either saying them outright or giving the impression that they are true successfully destroyed the book and its message.

I had a summer-long correspondence with the Food and Drug Administration that year, in which I sought from them their scientific proof that the CDC diet would not take off weight. Letters went back and forth for months. Mr. G. S. Goldhammer, who was director of the FDA Division of Regulatory Management, Bureau of Enforcement at that time, kept fobbing me off with references to material which, he said, proved the falseness of the CDC claims of success. In each case, I carefully read the reference and quoted it back to him, demonstrating that the very references he had given me confirmed the validity of the CDC diet. *Diets in which fat is restricted do not satisfy; where ample fat is allowed, the dieter eats less.*

When he could produce no more references, he finally wrote me, "In summation, if one follows the low calorie diet prescribed by Dr. Taller at one point in his book and disregards the contradictory statements made by Dr. Taller in other parts of his book to the effect that 'calories don't count,' etc., one might lose weight on the low calorie diet."

There is, of course, only one diet recommended in *Calories Don't Count*. It goes like this, in terms of menus:

Breakfast:

One or two eggs preferably scrambled in oil or margarine
One slice of gluten bread with cheese
Tea or coffee

Lunch:

Meat, fowl, fish or sea food (You must eat at least six
　to eight ounces)
Vegetables, chosen from a low carbohydrate list
One slice of gluten bread
Tea or coffee

Dinner:

Meat, fowl, fish or shellfish (At least 10 or 12 ounces.)
Low carbohydrate vegetable
One slice of gluten bread
Tea or coffee

Let's say you have two eggs for breakfast, plus one-fourth
pound of cheese. You have eight ounces of pork loin for
lunch plus a serving of green beans and a slice of bread. For
dinner you have a sirloin steak, weighing 12 ounces, plus a
serving of spinach and a slice of bread.

Then you are told you must somehow manage to consume three ounces of salad oil per day, plus two ounces of
margarine, which you can use any way you wish, like for
frying the eggs or melting over the vegetables or spreading
on the bread.

This amount of food for the day comes to 3935 calories.
Depending on the kind and amount of meat and cheese you
eat, the calories might be slightly lower or higher than that.
The usual reducing diet for women ranges from 1000 to
1400 calories per day, for men from 1400 to 1800 calories.
Can you tell me how the Food and Drug Administration
computes the CDC diet as "low calorie?"

They can't, of course, any more than you or I can. But
they have to get off the hook somehow; they have to dis-

credit this diet any way they can. So they say, hoping you won't ever check them on it, that what you end up with is in reality a low calorie diet. It isn't, as you can see from the above. The recommended diet is extremely high in calories. What happens is that you find you simply can't consume this much food—this kind of food, that is. It's just that simple. Your tongue, your appetite, your appestat, whatever it is that guides your eating habits and tells you when to shove your chair back, satisfied, simply prevents you from eating too much of this kind of diet.

Or, as *Stay Slim for Life* puts it, "On the 60 gram carbohydrate limitation the dieter must forego sugar, assorted pastries, pies, cakes, candy and all sweets. Fruits, fruit juices, cereals, potatoes, starchy vegetables and bread are all rigidly restricted. It doesn't take much detective work to account for the missing calories on the eat-all-you-want plan. You want only so much fat and protein, and you can't have sweets and starches. All those pleasure-giving foods which are left out lower the boom on calories."

What's wrong with that? Where is it written in the Book of Health that one must eat sweets or be unhealthy, that one must have desserts and sugary snacks all day long or be unhappy? Who said so, and how long have they been saying it? Only for the past couple of hundred years have we had access to this kind of food in any quantity at all. Are we to believe that somehow man managed to survive down through all the ages of time, eating food that was not nourishing him, was not pleasing him, made him unhappy? Try telling that to the Eskimos (among the happiest of people!) or the Masai or the many nations of people who have never tasted what we think of as desserts, pastries, candy and so forth, but who somehow manage to survive very happily, even though, let's face it, their mode of eating does not put much money into the coffers of the great food manufacturing companies.

It seems reasonable that many of Dr. Taller's patients found they simply could not eat as much as he told them to eat. It seems pretty obvious that a diet which brings forth such a criticism is quite a far cry from the average reducing diet. And it seems obvious that the reason for the success of the diet is the very fact which the title of the book tried to make clear but only managed to confuse still further: calories don't count. In other words, if you eat this way, you will not have to count calories.

The case of *Calories Don't Count* reached the halls of Congress in the fiery address of one knowledgeable congressman who called the FDA's attack on the book "Trial by press release." A well-known columnist who had reduced successfully and happily on the Taller diet took to the newspapers to champion its cause. An angry physician wrote to the *New England Journal of Medicine,* protesting the review of *CDC* which they had published, authored by Dr. Fredrick Stare of Harvard. He said, in part, "One might hope that Dr. Stare would give some commentary about the book and its contents, which have produced such amazing results, whatever validity the theory may have, despite its apparent contradiction of most accepted principles of weight reduction now used. It certainly deserves more than a brush-off!"

I think it does, too. And the reason is that the CDC diet is the same diet, in essence, that everyone referred to in this book has tested and recommends for excellent, sensible reasons which go far back into mankind's history on earth. These are all bona fide medical men, physicians, or research experts. They are not selling safflower oil or any other product. They are simply telling the truth, as their experiments

70

and research have shown it, and they are pinpointing carbohydrates—especially the highly concentrated, highly refined
carbohydrates—as the basic cause of our nation's enormous,
health-destroying cargo of overweight. They are also saying
that eating fat doesn't make you fat, because in a diet where
carbohydrates, especially refined carbohydrates, are sharply
restricted and protein is allowed in ample amounts, you
simply cannot eat too much fat. You don't want to. Furthermore, as time goes on, you no longer want the highly concentrated carbohydrates—the gooey desserts and the sticky
between-meal snacks. You are so well nourished that you
have mastered your addiction!

CHAPTER EIGHT

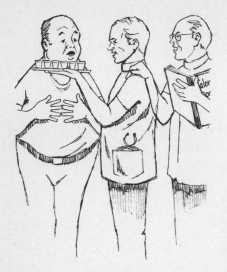

I CAN'T EAT THAT MUCH FOOD!

YOU WILL RECALL that the spokesman for the American Medical Association characterized Dr. Taller's book *Calories Don't Count* when it appeared as "ranking high on the list representing nutrition nonsense and food quackery." That was in 1962.

On October 5, 1964 the *Journal of the American Medical Association* printed an article by a group of researchers on obesity, at the University of Wisconsin Medical School. Headed by Dr. Edgar S. Gordon, this group of men had been reducing obese patients with a diet whose basis was six feedings daily of a high-protein, low-carbohydrate diet, *with considerable amounts of fat which were obligatory.* They gave the fat in the form of corn oil, cottonseed oil or safflower oil and their patients *had* to eat seven servings of fat every day. They complained about it, some of them. *It was too much food!*

Every patient was allowed the following foods every day: one egg, 11 ounces of meat, seven servings of fat, two cups of skim milk, two servings of fruit and vegetables (according to a list of allowed items) plus one-half slice of bread or its equivalent in carbohydrate. Does it sound familiar? It should, for this is basically the same diet recommended by Dr. Taller, with six small meals a day rather than three larger ones.

"Free foods" not limited in any way were artificially sweetened soft drinks, clear, fat-free broth, unsweetened plain gelatin or artificially-sweetened gelatin products, lemons, vinegar, spices and herbs. Alcoholic beverages were forbidden.

Dr. Gordon allows much more fruit than Dr. Taller allowed. His patients could have almost any fruit, provided the serving was small enough—that is, ½ a small banana, ½ cup orange juice, 2 medium dried prunes, and so forth. A taste, a nibble, no more. But a wider variety of fruits. Vegetables were essentially the same—the low carbohydrate ones. If his patients wanted to substitute one vegetable for their one-half slice of bread, they could. They could have, *instead—not in addition but instead* of the bread—one-half cup of beets, peas, pumpkin, carrots, squash, rutabaga, onions or turnips. Mid-morning and mid-afternoon snacks and a pre-bedtime snack consisted usually of 1 cup of skim milk plus one ounce of meat, or 2 ounces of meat.

Dr. Gordon's group had some other very interesting ideas on how such a program should begin. They fasted their patients for 48 hours, supposedly to pry them loose from whatever patterns of incorrect food metabolism had been bothering them. They started out on the diet fresh from a fast. Obese people, according to Dr. Gordon, behave metabolically like diabetics—they do not burn sugars normally, but dispose of them, instead, in fatty tissues. The fast, he said, changed this tendency toward a more normal one.

He went on to say that "an abundant supply of carbohydrate food exerts a powerful influence in directing the stream of glucose (sugar) metabolism into lipogenesis (fat formation), whereas a relatively low carbohydrate intake tends to minimize the storage of fat."

He goes on to say—and please keep in mind that this is being said in the sober and conservative pages of the *Journal of the American Medical Association* which had some months earlier castigated Dr. Taller as preaching nutritional nonsense—Dr. Gordon goes on to say, "Incorporation of a supplement of polyunsaturated fatty acid in the diet of human subjects has been found to accelerate the rate of oxidation of saturated or body fat." In easier words, if you take a certain amount of salad oil (rich in unsaturated fat) every day, this oil tends to melt away the excessive fat on your hips and thighs. "The exact mechanism of this effect remains unknown," says Dr. Gordon.

These are almost the exact words used by Dr. Taller to explain the necessity of taking safflower oil on his diet—the very words that brought down on his head the wrath of the FDA, the AMA and, finally, the court which, working on the premise that such a diet could not reduce anyone, declared that the Taller diet was a fraud and fined him heavily.

Yet the AMA is apparently convinced of the effectiveness of Dr. Gordon's diet. In a later issue (December 6, 1965) a doctor wrote asking whether this Gordon diet might be acceptable for diabetics—either those on oral drugs or insulin. Dr. Gordon himself answered this query. He said that the diet is indeed an excellent diet for obese diabetics as well as for obese non-diabetics. It's good for anyone!

Several months earlier, December 21, 1963, the *JAMA* printed an article by several Israeli physicians who were reducing out-patients at a clinic to which they came to eat a low-carbohydrate, high-protein diet totalling 1000 calories. The diet consisted of lean meat, fish, cottage cheese, eggs, soya flour (for vegetarians) yogurt, low carbohydrate vegetables, two portions of fruit and one slice of bread per day.

They state that almost none of their patients "cheated" by eating forbidden foods away from the clinic. "Another marked advantage. . . . is the effective re-education of dietary habits, such as eating a relatively full breakfast to forestall the pangs of hunger that lead to increased caloric intake."

Speaking of this aspect of the high protein diet, Dr. Gordon says, "One unexpected dividend that has emerged from the institution of this therapeutic program has been the spontaneous evolution of new and more beneficial dietary habits in a great many patients who have commented with great surprise about the apparent loss of old compulsions to eat and modification of cravings for certain high-carbohydrate foods."

They have overcome the addiction, you see, not by fasting, not by drugs, not by all kinds of extreme and heroic measures, but simply by returning to the kind of food human beings have eaten over millions of years, and eliminating the foods which have been introduced into our menus only within the past moment of time, speaking in terms of evolution.

Here are menus for a day on the Wisconsin diet. Sound familiar?

Breakfast

½ cup vitamin C-rich fruit (orange, grapefruit, tangerine or watermelon)
1 egg
1 ounce of meat—¼ cup
1 teaspoon margarine
½ slice of bread

Mid-Morning

1 cup skimmed milk
1 ounce of meat

Lunch

3 ounces of meat
vegetable from the allowed list-one or two cups
1 teaspoon margarine
6 teaspoons salad dressing on any salad vegetables

Mid-afternoon

2 ounces lean meat
½ cup skimmed milk

Dinner

3 ounces lean meat
allowed vegetables—one or two cups
6 teaspoons salad dressing on any salad vegetables
1 serving of fruit

Evening

½ cup skimmed milk
1 ounce of meat

76

The allowed vegetables are the ones whose carbohydrate content is five per cent or less. They are listed elsewhere in this book. The portions of fruit allowed are:

apple, one small, 2 inches
apple sauce—½ cup
apricots, dried—2 halves
       fresh—2 small
banana—½ small
blackberries—1 cup
blueberries—⅓ cup
raspberries—1 cup
strawberries—1 cup
cantaloupe—¼
cherries—10 large
dates—2
figs—1 small
grapefruit—½ small
grapes—12 large
orange—1 small
peach—1 medium
pineapple—½ cup
plums—2 medium
prunes—2 medium
raisins—2 tablespoons
tangerine—1 large
watermelon—1 cup

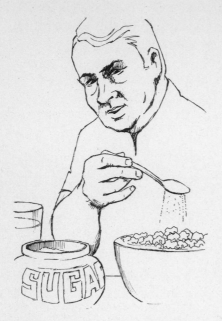

CHAPTER NINE

CUT DOWN, NOT OUT— IS THAT REALLY THE ANSWER?

THE AMERICAN Medical Association's official book on health for the layman—*Today's Health Guide*—devotes one chapter to Foods and Nutrition and one chapter to Obesity. There are 91 chapters in the book. This seems to show a careless lack of emphasis, since officially about 25 per cent of all Americans are thought to be overweight, from 11 to 45 per cent (in certain age groups) are thought to be obese. And, most important of all, since overweight is officially linked to such diseases as diabetes (3 million victims), heart conditions (12 million victims) arthritis (12 million victims) kidney disorders and many other disorders. This linkage could mean either that overweight is one of the causes of each of these disorders or that the same way of life which causes overweight also causes (at least in part) each of the other diseases.

However, the AMA seems to feel that the average American can eat what they call "a good well-rounded diet" since the right kind of food is readily available to almost all of us. Why, then, are millions of us overweight? Taking fewer calories than one needs seems within the capability of almost every person, writes the unnamed author of the chapter on obesity, yet "long-term observations indicate poor overall success for most 'dieters.' "

He goes on to list four aspects of the management of obesity: psychological, pharmaceutical, physical and dietary. That is, the person who overeats because of anxiety must see a psychiatrist or get "suitable guidance and support" from his doctor. As for drugs, the author states that they may for a time provide a "gimmick"—the element of magic for which the wavering will power inevitably reaches out. "However," he goes on, "they also serve as a crutch, detracting and diverting from the essential emphasis on dietary regulation. At best, they appear to afford only initial temporary help. They merely postpone the day when facts must be faced."

As for the physical management of overweight—exercise —there is a new approach to this, says the author. Where formerly we talked ourselves out of exercising by reminding ourselves that a 36-hour walk is required to shed just one pound of fat, someone has now figured out that taking one hour's walk every day for 36 days will accomplish the same result and will result in a loss of about 10 pounds in one year, which is certainly an achievement not to be despised. Furthermore, it has been shown that exercising does not increase the appetite correspondingly. That is, says this AMA author, your hour's walk every day will not result in such an increase in appetite that you will come home and eat enough to put on again every ounce you have lost. (As we have seen in other work along these lines, the evidence strongly suggests that the more exercise you get, the more easily is your appetite regulated to just that amount of food which you need. The AMA book does not mention these experiments.)

On the dietary aspects of reducing, the AMA book has a number of surprisingly sensible things to say. "It is generally agreed that given adequate determination, weight can be lost on virtually any dietary plan, good or bad, that insures a caloric intake less than what is required by the energy used. It is equally apparent that many diets are only temporarily effective and do not promote the fundamental purpose of permanent loss, not to mention good eating habits."

So any diet that results in your eating fewer calories will bring about loss of weight. But it should also be a diet that embodies good eating habits which will stay with you for life, not just for the duration of the diet period. This automatically eliminates most of the "fad" diets. Says our author.

"The diet should be balanced and complete in conformity with the Recommended Dietary Allowance of the National Research Council. Only the physician can assure the dieter on this point." This appears to indicate that only a physician is qualified to tell you how to include in every day's meals the four food groups which are officially recommended for nutritious diet: the meat, fish, poultry group, the milk, eggs and cheese group, the fruit and vegetable group and the cereal group. This doesn't appear to present such an insurmountably difficult problem to most adults, it seems to us. But apparently the AMA feels that only a doctor is capable of understanding and explaining these categories.

And one aspect of the problem of overweight for most of us is that far too much of our food intake is not included in any of these four food groups, but comes to us loaded with calories and spiked with appetizing taste whether natural or synthetic. We refer, of course, to those foods which consist mostly of sugar: sugar itself dumped into coffee, tea or cereals (50 calories for 2 rounded teaspoons), soft drinks (137 calories in 12 ounces) fruit flavored soda (161 calories in 12 ounces) a chocolate bar (290 calories in a 2-ounce bar), and of course all those luscious desserts which may contain some small excuse in the form of fruit or protein but which contain so much sugar that they bear no relation to the relative amounts of sugar found in natural foods like fruits. A slice of cherry pie, for instance, contains 340 calories. An entire cup of fresh raw cherries contains only 65. The cherry pie contains 55 grams of carbohydrate. The raw cherries contain 15 grams.

The AMA book goes at some length into the subject of calories and diets—recommending that protein calories should account for 12 to 20 per cent of the diet total, fat calories should contribute 25 to 30 per cent, but maybe, they say, 45 to 50 per cent is a better plan considering "the appetite-satisfying and energy values of fat." The total carbohydrate count in calories should be from 40 to 60 per cent of the total and it should provide "sufficient fiber content (roughage) for normal bowel function and to sustain useful intestinal bacteria."

Using just this last criterion, we can cross off the sugar in coffee and tea, soft drinks of all kinds, candy of all kinds, chewing gum, and most prepared desserts for the simple reason that none of these contain any fiber at all which is likely to take care of the body functions mentioned above. This leaves us with vegetables and fruits as the only acceptable carbohydrate part of our diet, along with cereals. How much fiber or roughage is present in cereal foods would depend, it is obvious, on how they have been processed. Certainly whole grain flours contain far more fiber than refined white ones. Whole grain cereals of all kinds contain far more fiber than the puffed, flaked, highly processed breakfast cereals. The bran which many people take to prevent constipation is simply one part of the wheat which has been removed in refining and milling.

One final word from the AMA. They stress the great value of the regular timing of meals. "These, whatever their number, should be consumed at regular, though not necessarily equal intervals. Meal schedules should be set and followed consistently seven days a week. Only in this manner can the rhythmic pattern be developed that is essential for a long-term adherence to a reducing and especially a maintenance regimen."

Here are some of the recommendations made in the chapter on nutrition. Milk and milk products can improve the value of every meal. In case you object to actually drinking milk, equivalent amounts of protein and minerals are available from cheese (a one-inch cube of cheddar is equivalent to ⅔ cup of milk). In the meat group—that is, foods high in protein—the author includes nuts, peas and beans because they contribute essentially the same nutrients as meat and fish: protein, iron, and the B vitamins largely. "It is recommended that some meat, poultry, fish or eggs be eaten at each meal. Eggs (two for a serving), dry beans, dry peas and lentils (1 cup, cooked, per serving), peanut butter (4 tablespoons), and nuts can be used in place of one serving of meat when menu variety is desired."

They recommend luncheon meats, hamburgers, hot dogs and the inexpensive cuts of meat if you are keeping a tight budget. Of vegetables and fruits they say: "Vegetables and fruits are the foods most frequently neglected by children and young people . . . Your diet should include four or more servings from vegetable-fruit groups every day." Of course it is generally well known that at least one of these should be a food high in vitamin C, citrus probably, and one a food high in vitamin A. (That is, a bright yellow or green food.)

Here is a paragraph which seems to us highly controversial, yet it is quietly glossed over as if it were a well-proven scientific fact. Says the AMA author, "The preferred way to reduce weight is to cut down on the amount of food consumed. One should cut *down*, however, not cut *out*. Many people have the mistaken notion that some foods are fattening and should be avoided; this is not so. No one food can be considered fattening because each food contributes a certain percentage of the day's calories. The true cause of overweight is the total amount of food calories one consumes per day."

This one paragraph, it seems to us, begs the entire question and leaves the average modern American still adrift on a sea of confusion in regard to what food brought him to his present unhappy state of overweight. "Cut *down,* not *out.*" So should we have only one chocolate bar and one teaspoon of sugar in coffee instead of two, one doughnut instead of three, two cokes instead of four and so on? But acting on this same recommendation, we will also have only one hamburger instead of two, one egg instead of two, one chicken leg instead of two, one glass of milk instead of two.

So the average person whose bad eating habits have brought him to a condition of overweight will now probably cut his protein and fat allotment in half along with his carbohydrate allotment. Yet there is no evidence anywhere in medical literature that protein *per se* is fattening, no matter how much one eats of it. The reason seems to be that we have a built-in control over the amount of high-protein foods that are acceptable to our appetite and our desires for food. And there is convincing evidence that many modern foods high in carbohydrate tend to be far more fattening than even their high calorie content would indicate, because they tend to make addicts out of people who consume them every day.

We all know people who just can't get by without their mid-morning and mid-afternoon cokes. We all know people who go on chocolate bar binges as alcoholics go on lost weekends. They just can't stop. We all know people who have started to add a sweet bun to their breakfast, a piece of pie to their lunch, a snack of ice cream and cookies before bed. And they just can't do without these treats, to say nothing of mints to suck between meals and a daily pack of chewing gum, each stick of which gives a pleasant sweet taste for 15 minutes or so.

Cutting down on protein and fat, cutting in half one's allotment of fresh fruits and vegetables by cutting "down, not out" is quite likely to bring below the recommended level the amount of several very important nutrients which may be marginal in many peoples' diets, anyway. Certainly the individual who has well-sugared coffee and doughnuts for breakfast, hamburger, potato chips and coffee for lunch should not be told to "cut down" on his intake of fruits and vegetables since he doesn't seem to be eating enough of these foods to keep him in reasonably good health, as it is. Once you get a taste for desserts, pastries and goodies from the bakery you usually find plain vegetables and fruits rather dull. So at dinner, appalled at having lost no ounce of weight that day, he may decide to eat only half as much of carrots or salad or potato, along with, of course, half as much dessert. (He's cutting *down*, not cutting *out* anything.)

How much more sensible it would seem to counsel dropping all those foods which are not included in the basic four groups. Then even if you cut *down* on some of these foods you would not be so likely to shortchange yourself on vitamins and minerals, because you would be eating more of the basic four. The major official objection to foods like soft drinks, candy and desserts has always been a very sound one—that they satiate the appetite very quickly and leave one with little appetite for "the basic four" groups of food. Yet their staying power is so short that one soon needs more food. And this food is likely to be more of the same.

"You'll spoil your dinner with that candy" is not just an old wives' tale. The child who has been nibbling on candy or pouring down soft drinks most of the day will probably not be interested in eating meat, vegetables and fruit when he sits down with the family for dinner. How can he?

And how can he possibly be completely nourished, when the sweets he has been stuffing all day long, which destroy his appetite for dinner, consist almost entirely of what are called "empty calorie" foods contributing nothing whatever that food is supposed to contain, except pure carbohydrate, which translates into pure calories and nothing else.

Nowhere in official and especially medical thinking about overweight and the problem of staying on a reducing diet do we find any recognition of the fact that such foods are not essential to either good health or delightful eating. A craving for them represents, in essence, a perversion of true appetite, an addiction. By completely eliminating such foods, the addiction can be cured, as any other addiction can be cured. And once there is no more craving for such foods, the appetite mechanism settles down and becomes what it started out to be hundreds of thousands of years ago—a proper guide, a reliable guide, to how much to eat. And problems of obesity disappear painlessly and forever.

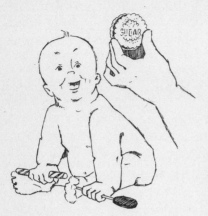

CHAPTER TEN

IT'S BABY FAT. HE'LL OUTGROW IT

Here are some quotes from articles in my file on fat children and adolescents:

"The problem of overweight is one of the most puzzling mysteries confronting the medical profession today. . . . the more we learn about its various aspects, the more confusing is the role of the physician."

"Investigators are astounded by their own statistics which suggest that already at least 10,000,000 young people up to nineteen may be affected by overweight."

"In one study, 23 per cent of the girls and almost 36 per cent of the boys were overweight. Dr. Jean Mayer of Harvard, acknowledged as one of the world's leading authorities on juvenile obesity, estimates that 15 to 20 per cent of all adolescents are heavy enough to be classed as full-fledged medical problems." (But the doctors don't know what made them fat. It's a medical mystery.)

"Some families serve rich food constantly without regard to nutritional requirements. In other households, regular meals have gone by the board because of the family's irregular hours. . . . Youngsters fail to get full-balanced meals, filling up with rich snacks instead. Snacks, largely in the form of sweets of all kinds, are also doled out as supplements to meals . . . they have become a ritualized part of the movies and are inseparably associated with TV viewing."

"Recent studies with laboratory animals show that diets with a high sugar content stimulate the animals to eat more and to deposit more fat than diets in which starch is the chief carbohydrate."

"If children are given a wide variety of foods, they're less likely to focus on those high-calorie foods that create obesity."

"It's no wonder that pediatrics is plagued these days by a condition very discouraging and hard to do anything about —juvenile obesity. When I went into pediatrics 40 years ago, the opposite condition, undernutrition, plagued us, but it did offer some chance of medical correction. Obesity cannot be corrected medically. It requires self-discipline. And where is there any of that today?"

"Family eating patterns are deeply ingrained. Mothers of fat children are invariably excellent cooks and overly concerned about the adequacy of their offsprings' diet. They undermined the adolescent's efforts to lose weight by excessive baking or by forcing them to help with the food preparation. . . ."

"The parent may actually be unaware that she is . . . overstuffing the child. She will say 'He doesn't eat anything but he gains weight.' What she really means is that he doesn't eat breakfast (a common pattern among obese youngsters) but there is an increasing crescendo of eating as the day goes by."

"By the time the girls have finished a session at the camp for fatties . . . sessions on nutrition have made them experts at devising *a sound, high-protein, moderate-fat, low-carbohydrate diet.*"

In many of the articles quoted above, the authors—doctors and non-doctors alike—put forward every conceivable reason for childhood obesity, except the one that is staring them in the face: the change in the character of American food, within the past 30 years or so.

They announce that they are unable to understand juvenile obesity. The more they learn about it the less they understand it. Medical and scientific journals are crammed with careful laboratory studies in which volunteers ate measured amounts of fats, proteins and carbohydrates, were weighed every hour, were exercised, talked to, watched—all to no avail. The results seemed to show all kinds of contradictions.

The children inherited their tendency to obesity. But on the other hand, perhaps they did not. Their mothers were good cooks; the mothers never learned to cook, hence the children had to eat snacks. Fat children don't eat as much as thin children; on the other hand, fat children tend to eat no breakfast and then to go on stuffing themselves at an accelerating rate the rest of the day. The contradictions pile on the contradictions!

What would you think of a researcher who decided to study the cause of automobile accidents by taking apart a last-century buggy and carriage? He studies the physiology and anatomy of the horse. Then he places a volunteer in a horse and buggy outfit and tests his reactions to moving about in this contraption. Could such a procedure conceivably throw any light on today's incidence of automobile accidents?

Today, gentlemen, we have the automobile, remember, which has replaced the horse and buggy. We should therefore abandon research having to do with the horse and buggy, and study the entirely different circumstances brought to highway travel by the automobile. Isn't this the sensible, in fact, the only way to make any kind of scientific study of automobile accidents? I think we would all agree that it is.

But where diet is concerned, researchers are still poking around in the last century, dealing with such ancient concepts as how many calories will be used up in running a mile, with apparently no inkling that the situation in regard to food today is as different from the last generation, physiologically speaking, as the automobile is different from the horse and buggy.

Most children today get their first taste of pure sugar—a substance that exists nowhere in nature—long before they are weaned. By the time they are in kindergarten, candy and soft drinks are considered as important a part of their diet as meat and milk. Do you know any child who has not been fed candy before weaning time? Do you know any grade school child who does not drink a given number of soft drinks every week, if not every day?

Have you sat in restaurants and watched children order cokes and french fried potatoes for lunch while their parents smile and urge them to have dessert? Have you ever attended a children's party and measured the amount of pure sugar consumed by each tiny toddler present?

Unless there is some recognition of what has happened to food in the last 30 years, our researchers will never get any nearer to solving the puzzle of obesity than they are today. It is not the same food it always has been, gentlemen. It's a different thing, entirely—as different as the automobile is different from the horse and buggy.

Those of us who are forty years or older grew up in a time when there were sweets, of course. But they were treats! You had them at Christmas and Easter, or maybe on Saturday afternoon. You ate ice cream on Sundays, mostly. Baking a cake or a batch of cookies was a long detailed process. These things weren't available everywhere you turned, inexpensive, attractive, wrapped to take out, enclosed in coin machines.

Put in its simplest form, many children have become addicts to a drug—sugar and, to some extent, starch, two foods which have been denuded of the fiber and food elements that accompany them in food. It's just that simple. Remember what Dr. Cleave and Dr. Yudkin said? So long as food retains to a large extent its natural character, it also contains a built-in guarantee against overeating. You can't eat enough raw apples to make you fat. They have a built-in guarantee. But you can eat many times that much sugar in candy bars without ever knowing when to stop eating! And the sugar makes you fat. The apples don't.

Why is this such a difficult concept for our learned researchers to grasp? Partly, we suspect, as Dr. Cleave says, because it's too simple. Modern researchers, delighting in all the abstruse complexity of the modern physiology laboratory, just couldn't possibly grasp an idea of such abject simplicity—that as soon as you stop *concentrating the carbohydrates in food, you will recreate in Western human beings the ability to know when to stop eating*. It will be automatic. And so long as you continue to feed people food which deranges this appestat, if that's what you want to call it, you will have widespread obesity.

90

The fault lies not in indulgent parents, in over-protective mothers and silly grandmothers, not in psychiatrically deranged and emotionally disturbed children. The fault lies in the kitchens of the great food manufacturing companies from whence, we are told, some 12,000 "new products" will have emerged in the next few years—to complete the destruction of the American appestat. For all the millions of years of evolution, remember, human taste buds and human tongues have had no experience with "food" like this. Why is it so surprising that there should be a nation-wide reaction of total inability to cope with such a new environmental element within the space of only a few years? What other reaction could there possibly be?

One other fault lies in the modern love for specialties. Today all scientists are specialists. The man who develops the flavor for the new breakfast "tart" knows nothing about obesity and its causes. He's a specialist in flavors. The men who invent the new soft drink know nothing about overweight. They are specialists in such things as viscosity of fluids, and the dissolving rates of sugars and the mixtures of dyes that may produce pleasing colors.

On the other hand, the doctor who treats obesity knows nothing or next to nothing about modern food. Tell him that we will have 12,000 new items in every supermarket within a few years and he will think this is fine, because it will never occur to him that this will be any different from what food has always been—something composed of fats, proteins, carbohydrates and sundry other things like vitamins and minerals in a well-ordered balance, as nature has been dishing them out for millions of years. Unless or until he gets into a kitchen or a factory and sees how today's food is put together, he will never know that when he tells his patients to "cut down on calories" and eat less, he is being about as effective as if he were to put a 19th century farm lad down in the middle of an expressway in a high-powered racing car and say to him, "Drive carefully, son."

So we end this discussion of childhood obesity, surely one of the most widespread tragedies of our time, foreboding a future nation with ever-higher incidence figures of diabetes, heart trouble, circulatory trouble and all the other related conditions, with the quote we gave earlier: "the girls at a summer camp for fatties became expert by the end of the summer in devising a sound, high-protein, moderate-fat, low-carbohydrate diet." This seems to be the most helpful note sounded in all the literature on childhood obesity.

Children should be told, from the time they can understand words, that they may have all they want to eat of certain foods, none at all of others. They must eat at least three meals a day, preferably more. All the food eaten must not contain more than a given number of carbohydrate units a day. And these units must be from fruits, vegetables, nuts, and grains. We could wipe out childhood obesity in a few years.

The youngsters would then know when to stop eating. They would never know the pathological hunger that goes along with teenage "reducing diets." They would never know the apathy, the irritability, the restlessness, the fatigue, the lack of interest that goes along with low blood sugar levels at 10 in the morning and four in the afternoon. Children brought up on sugar are starving children! Children who go off to school without breakfast, then eat a skimpy lunch and come ravenous to the dinner table are starving children. It's no wonder they overeat. It's no wonder they get fat.

Listen to what one anthropologist at the Public Health Service had to say approximately ten years ago about the food habits of your children and the kinds of food they are offered:

"In a typical emporium of one (supermarket) chain, I recently counted, all on open counters, the varieties and sizes of packaged or boxed candies and nuts (no cookies) excluding candy bars, gums, suckers and rolls of mints, with a price range from about 25 cents to $3. The number shocked me: 172. The varieties of candy bars, gums, and "mints" (excluding cough drops) sold separately, not in boxes, numbered 106. . . . . A large and typical drugstore in another chain was similarly surveyed the same week. It had 135 packaged or boxed candies and nuts and 103 bars, chewing-gums, and mints. The price range of this class of goods was 4 cents to 15 cents, within the reach— literally and figuratively—of nearly every child.

"In our apparently rich culture, part of the range of choice is illusory and misleading. We are not nutritionally much better off for having three kinds of lettuce on sale at the same time in the same store . . . It is more important for a child to choose between a candy bar and an apple— *and to have both equally available and tempting*—than for him to choose among 12 chocolate bars, in reality choosing only between a gold wrapper and a silver wrapper. . . .

"Nutritionists are united, I suppose, in believing and saying that children should eat less of the sweets, certainly that they should not consume them to the exclusion of more protective foods. There are various ways that this might be done, but probably won't be. We have seen how our technology, economic abundance, customs and values involved in merchandising and consumer purchasing are related to dietary habits. So one way of decreasing sugary goodies would be to control at the source. This might be undertaken in some countries but it will not be in this one. The reformers would have to 'take on' the soft drink, confectionery, and baking industries; and. . . . the first two alone constitute two billion dollars worth of wholesale business. With the food industry stand the paper and packaging industries, the importers of sugar and chocolate, and various lesser ones that together can be powerful.

"Then there is the advertising business, which would have to change an important part of the content of advertising. In 1957, the total volume of advertising, including newspapers, magazines, radio and television and direct mail cost $10,310,600,000. . . . . any industry so massive and with so many specialized parts and strong connections is almost impossible to move."

If you are seriously and conscientiously going on the high-protein, medium-fat, low-carbohydrate diet, chances are that you can take as many pounds off your overweight child as you take off yourself, with no more effort than choosing your purchases wisely at the supermarket, and laying down a few immutable rules for how the entire family will eat from this time on. *Everyone will eat breakfast*. If this means missing the entire late show, or late party or late dance, so be it. Everyone in the family must get up in time to eat a high protein breakfast. *That's the rule from now on*.

The breakfast consists of high protein foods, nothing more. Meat, poultry, fish, eggs, cheese, milk can be eaten for breakfast in any quantity, in any way, in any recipe. Nothing else may be eaten except fruit. You can easily manage this by just seeing to it that there isn't any other kind of food in the house. At lunch the same rules prevail. If you pack lunch for the children or anyone else in the family, the high-protein, low-carbohydrate rule prevails. If the children eat lunch at school your work will be harder, but you may be pleasantly surprised to find that, after a time, they are just naturally selecting more nutritious food from the school menu. The coke-french-fry lunches won't be nearly so appealing somehow. For snacks you will provide any kind of nuts, popcorn, fruit in abundance, cheese, raw vegetables. For beverages, milk, vegetable juices or fruit juices.

If the adults in your family are eating this way, it's remarkable how soon the children will find their way happily along the same path. Of course if the adults continue to stuff themselves with sugar, desserts, soft drinks, sticky buns, pastries and candy, the children will follow suit. Why not? Didn't they learn most of their habits—good and bad—from you?

CHAPTER ELEVEN

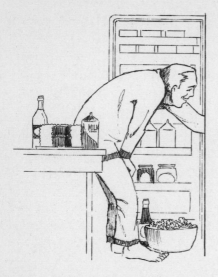

HOW OFTEN AND HOW SHOULD YOU EAT?

I F YOU WANTED to select several characteristic ways of eating that seem to appear oftener than any other in surveys of overweight and obese individuals they are these: they tend to skimp on food early in the day, then eat huge meals in the evening. Many of them go right on eating all evening and some of them get up at night to raid the refrigerator. And they tend to eat fast, very fast.

Time and time again you read that the person of average or normal weight, the fellow who seemingly has no weight problem at all eats a big breakfast, high in protein, may have a glass of milk or juice at coffee break, eats a commendably nutritious lunch and a dinner that is very moderate so far as courses and content go. Chances are he has no desire for food in the evening.

The overweight individual complains that he has a problem that can't be solved. Look at the thin people! They eat big breakfasts and lunches, while he starves himself! It must be that they have been endowed by providence with a special metabolism that never allows them to gain unwanted weight, while he, the victim of some merciless god, cannot lose weight no matter how he starves himself. These days many young folks especially seem beset with eating patterns that presage possible disaster in later years.

They omit breakfast entirely or they snatch an inadequate breakfast on the way out the door. Why? They say it's because they don't have time to eat. They got up too late, or they just aren't hungry in the morning, or nobody ever prepares breakfast for them or they don't like to eat alone or any of a host of other reasons—all of which could be fairly easily remedied if their parents paid half as much attention to what their children were eating as they do to other much less important aspects of family life.

So, many kids are off to school with perhaps four hours ahead of the hardest kind of work and no food to provide energy for this work. Blood sugar is usually at its lowest level when we get out of bed. Four more hours without food will almost guarantee that the blood sugar will plunge even farther down. If there's time for snacks at school, chances are they will be something sugary. "It gives quick energy," you know.

The overweight child may try to get by with little or no lunch. Trying to starve himself, you see, so that the kids won't call him fatty. By the time school is out, hunger pangs, headache, fatigue, faintness will win out. Gorging time is here. This is the pattern that brings on what the obesity specialists call the "night-eating syndrome."

How much does it have to do with our present-day problems of obesity and overweight? Look at it in the light of evolution. It seems likely that human beings, from earliest times of recorded history and before that, ate when they were hungry and/or when there was food available. Nowhere in history, or in the science of nutrition or dietetics is there any law which says that human beings should eat only three times a day or twice a day or once a day. We probably guide ourselves by three meals a day in this country mostly because it's convenient for the cook. In other countries, two meals are standard, or four or five.

Doesn't it seem reasonable that early man, hunting or gathering food, ate whenever he found something edible? He had no way to preserve it and chances are he was hungry much of the time. Even after he settled down in communities, because he had discovered how to plant cereals and grains which could be stored for winter eating, there wasn't much chance that he would overeat, for food was still remarkably scarce, and physical work extremely hard.

In this context, then, listen to some recent findings in regard to the damage you may be doing yourself by omitting or skimping on some meals and trying to make up for it in one or two big meals.

From the *American Journal of Clinical Nutrition,* May, 1966, evidence from a Czechoslovakian study that boys and girls in boarding schools gained weight when they ate three meals a day, did not gain weight when they ate *the same food in five smaller meals a day.*

From the National Institute of Arthritis and Metabolic Diseases, studies showing that animals eating only once or twice a day had more susceptibility to diabetes, high cholesterol levels in their blood and obesity, than animals that nibbled all day long.

From the University of Virginia Medical School, May 4, 1963, a report that rats which were "trained" to eat within a two-hour period *consumed more food in that time than*

98

fellow-rats which were permitted to eat all day long—nibble, that is. Dr. William Parson who conducted the research, said that about 60 per cent of all fat people eat only one big meal a day, perhaps skipping breakfast, skimping on lunch and fasting between meals. He has found, he says, that periods of "starvation" have been shown to alter the chemical content of fatty tissue. *The rats which ate only during the two-hour allotted time became overweight. Those which nibbled all day did not.*

Proceedings of the Nutrition Society, Volume 26, No. 2, 1967, reported that studies on 900 individuals of different ages revealed that a pattern of three or fewer meals a day (as compared to more frequent intake of smaller meals— five or more a day) led to a tendency to overweight. In elderly men there was also an increase in cholesterol levels in the blood and a tendency toward diabetic blood sugar levels. The authors warn that the average person today uses less energy in physical work, consumes relatively enormous amounts of sugar and is becoming increasingly accustomed to postponing his main evening meal!

The authors ask whether it may not be possible that adaptive mechanisms that developed during man's long struggle for food and life may become unhealthful under conditions prevailing today. Ten thousand years ago the fellow who killed a deer may have stuffed himself with the prospect of going hungry until he came upon another game animal to kill. There was just no way to preserve the meat —he had to stuff himself! But think of the physical exertion it took to find the next piece of meat and to make the next killing!

From the *British Medical Journal,* April 16, 1968, comes a report of treating "refractory obesity" with five meals a day—very small meals, it is true—but five of them a day!

The purpose was to "avoid long fasts" and to give food often enough and in sufficient quantity to prevent or relieve hunger and yet to restrict calories. Fourteen dieters took off an average of about 10 pounds in three months on this diet. These people were "obese"—that is, at least 20 per cent overweight. They were given a list of over 70 "meals" or "snacks," whichever you prefer to call them. Each meal contained only about 200 calories, making a total of 1000 calories a day.

Here were some of the snacks: ½ grapefruit and 1 slice of bread; clear soup with vegetables (2 ounces); five ounces of meat with low starch vegetables; one ounce of lean bacon and one fried egg; cold meat plus salad and fruit. And so forth.

In *Nutrition Today,* volume 1, 1966, Dr. Jean Mayer of Harvard suggested that the person who cannot stick to a reducing diet because he is actually experiencing hunger pangs should be advised to time his eating to periods of peak hunger—this may mean eliminating "meals" and substituting "snacks."

In his excellent book, *Overweight,* Dr. Mayer tells us that just exposing laboratory rats to food once a day instead of all day increased their capacity *to make fat,* although they did not eat more. Chickens, too, fed only once a day, become "a little fatter."

There is a lot more such evidence available in scientific and medical literature if you're interested in searching for it. But why not just relax and accept it? Surely it isn't an insurmountable hardship for anyone to space his eating so that he never gets really terribly hungry. With food available almost everywhere you go today, it's possible to "snack" almost anywhere, almost any time of day.

If you choose the snacks carefully, the result may be to

straighten out your disordered mechanism for handling food and to ease your hunger at regular mealtime, so that you just won't have any urge to overeat. If you choose the wrong snacks, the result could be total disaster.

It's here that people who know absolutely nothing about nutrition can steer you so terribly wrong. Recently a psychologist wrote a book on how to reduce, which got a big play on TV, radio and in women's magazines. Deeply immersed in psychological theories as she was, this lady had it all figured out that the reason people can't take off weight is their psychological craving for something sweet! Her solution—a lollipop every couple of hours! Along with that a diet so bereft of anything nutritious that it's just bound to produce not only pathological hunger but perhaps florid vitamin and mineral deficiency, if you stick with it long enough.

But quite apart from nutritional deficiency, just think what the unbuffered sugar of a lollipop (sucked slowly for as long as you can make it last) three or four times a day is going to do to your teeth! The prospect is so horrendous that we wonder the entire dental profession didn't rise up in horror and denounce this outrage!

Then, in the light of what we have just learned about blood sugar regulation and the absolute necessity for eating sugar *only in complex combinations with protein, fat and other food elements,* just think of all that straight sugar going down three or four times a day—and imagine what it's going to do to your sugar-regulating mechanism!

The diet counsels you against fat: you can eat a pancake for breakfast with syrup but no butter! You can eat a hamburger but only if you carefully pat off all the fat it contains. You must use buttermilk and skim milk. Then, for Sunday evening dinner, you are told to eat *nothing but an entire pint of "dietetic ice cream" which means ice cream made with a sugar substitute.* Ice cream can contain up to 16 per cent fat. So your body mechanisms for dealing with fat, which you have been starving, disrupting and torturing all week, are suddenly confronted with a full pint—two cups—of fatty stuff all at once. It is hard to imagine any less physiological or sensible thing to do. Then, of course, at ten Sunday evening, you have your usual lollipop so that the sugar stays in your mouth, around your teeth and scouting around in your poor, nearly empty stomach all night!

If you are counting carbohydrate units—and we assume you are—then these must, of course, be included in your snacks, as well as your meals. The object of the whole endeavor is to spread the eating out over the day—*but to eat no more than you have been eating at one, two or three meals. And to eat only foods high in protein and low in starch and sugar*—especially the quickly assimilated sugars such as are found in candy, pastries, desserts and soft drinks chiefly.

It's perfectly possible to carry high protein snacks with you and it's possible to find high protein snacks almost any place you might be these days. Have a cheese sandwich rather than a doughnut, and leave the bread on the plate. Or order a dish of cottage cheese. Many supermarkets now sell tiny, one-serving cans of tuna and salmon which can be eaten as a snack, slowly and appreciatively. There's no carbohydrate there, so you needn't count. The cans are as easy to carry as a compact or a key case.

A hard-boiled egg will fit into anybody's pocket or purse and will keep well for an entire day. It will come out at snack time looking fresh and appetizing, if you wrap it in a sandwich bag. The same goes for a piece of cheese—almost any cheese. And are you going to be sitting around the coffee-break table at the office craving the chocolate bar and the sticky bun someone else is eating? Perhaps, just at first. But you're going to be very surprised at how soon the egg or the piece of cheese looks much more appetizing than the candy bar or the sticky bun! And you will find that the egg or the cheese stays with you, right with you, stilling hunger pangs and stomach butterflies until lunch time.

Will people think you're peculiar? Do you care? If you do, then tell them your doctor said you must eat this way.

Once you have established the habit of the high protein diet and the habit of taking high protein snacks throughout the day, you may find that you do not want food before bedtime. For older folks especially, this may be a great blessing, for there is considerable evidence that food before bedtime may result in insomnia, due to problems with ageing digestive tracts. If you still feel hungry before bedtime, then the snack must be high-protein—no doughnuts, no soft drinks, no cake.

One of the great nutrition experts on obesity of our time once remarked that he had never seen a grossly overweight person who did not eat fast. I have watched carefully since I read this and I have never seen an overweight person who did not eat fast. Furthermore, I have noticed that the kind of thin people who appear to be able to eat anything they want without putting on any unwanted weight eat slowly, so slowly that they are usually the last person finished with a meal. They find it impossible to "grab a sandwich" at a coffee bar while they are trying to make a bus, because they simply can't get the food down fast enough.

All their lives they have eaten slowly. They allow for this. They get up early enough in the morning so they can linger over breakfast. They never arrange for a lot of activities during an hour lunch period so they will have to rush through lunch. They *can't* rush through lunch. They must have time to eat.

Part—and an important part—of the digestive process takes place in the mouth. The food must be mixed sufficiently with saliva to bring about some of the chemical changes that must take place before this same food can be properly handled by the digestive juices in the lower part of the digestive tract. If you swallow it whole, this process simply can't take place.

You are going to be eating a different kind of food from now on—a kind of food that *needs* more chewing. Nobody has to chew a piece of cake, or a dish of commercial cereal, or a doughnut. All the fiber has been taken out of foods like this and they have a tendency to melt in your mouth, leaving you no reason to chew. Meat, fish, cheese, poultry, fruits and vegetables must be chewed. Chew them. Linger over them. Make them last as long as you can, every mouthful.

CHAPTER TWELVE

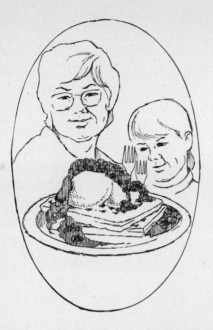

"BUT I INHERIT MY TENDENCY TO OVER- WEIGHT!"

D<small>O YOU?</small> Or do you inherit the eating patterns, menu-planning and meal-spacing of your family, the recipes of your great-grandmother who baked the best pies in the county, or the family tradition that "everybody's fat in this family because we have a sweet tooth and besides you need lots of sugar for energy?"

There doesn't seem to be any scientific way to decide this issue: whether one can inherit the tendency to overweight, regardless of what one eats. There seems to be no way of separating one from the other, without confining the subjects in locked rooms and doling out their food, as one would with laboratory animals. But people are not laboratory animals and eating patterns may have something to do with every bit of family lore and community culture that we have picked up along life's road.

(But somehow we can't stop thinking about those many

groups and nations of people who—unhealthy in many ways because of lack of hygiene and other amenities—still don't ever become fatties no matter what their grandparents did, *so long as they go on eating their natural diets high in protein and low in carbohydrate with no access to refined carbohydrates.* And, somehow, as soon as they begin to eat "civilized" food, they begin to put on weight, regardless of how splendidly thin and lissome all their ancestors were!)

It is believed that diabetics inherit a tendency to diabetes, that is, the child with one diabetic parent is more likely to be diabetic than the child of non-diabetics. The child of two diabetic parents has far more chances of being a diabetic than either of the two aforementioned ones. And most specialists in obesity seem to believe that the tendency to overweight is inherited.

Obesity and Health, published by the Public Health Service in 1966, states, "reports from studies of human populations strongly suggest the existence of a hereditary factor. . . . Studies of adopted children show that their weight bears little relation to the weight of their foster parents even if the children are adopted at birth . . ."

What about that ubiquitous "sweet tooth" that we keep blaming our eating habits on? All of us have it. Even the Eskimos prepare what they think is a great delicacy—a kind of ice cream made from seal fat and little berries that grow in their far north land during the summer. Thinking in terms of evolution, let's suppose for a moment that the part of our tongues which registers "sweet, oh, that tastes good!" developed over millions of years in response to fruits and berries that were available, along with occasional honeycombs and possibly flowers which contain nectar—all of them sweet to some extent.

Doesn't it seem possible that we evolved, *needing the*

nutrients that come along with the sweet taste in such foods? Human beings are almost alone among animals in their requirement for vitamin C. Almost all other animals make their own. But we must have a certain small amount of this highly perishable vitamin in our food or we die of scurvy. It occurs in nature mostly in fresh fruits, berries, stems and leaves—the juicy delights that taste sweet. Some B vitamins, vitamin A and many minerals are in these same foods. So as our ancestors, many generations back, threaded their way through woods, meadows, grasslands, eating anything that came along, doesn't it seem possible that the sweet taste guided them to foods that were essential for good health? Or, to put it another way, doesn't it seem possible that we evolved liking sweet things because they were inextricably bound up with things that were good for us? Over millions of years, we thus could be said to have developed a need, a craving, *for the things that go along with the sweet taste.*

Today, our tongues, trained over the centuries to respond positively to a sweet taste, keep telling us "This is good, this is nourishing, eat plenty of this," when we encounter the sweet taste in food. And, if we were still finding wild apples and plums growing on forest trees, if we were still searching the thickets for wild raspberries and the meadows for wild strawberries, this age-old, slowly evolved protective mechanism would still be functioning as it was meant to function, leading us to foods that we need and turning us aside from foods that taste bad or bitter.

We never outgrow our need *for the nutrients that, in nature, go along with the sweet taste.* But today, food technologists know how to separate the sweet taste entirely from everything else that is in the natural food: protein, vitamins and minerals being the chief nutrients we are most familiar with. They present you with something like a soft drink which pleases that part of your tasting apparatus that registers "sweet," but they have not included in this "food" any of the things our ancestors obtained when they followed their "sweet tooth" to fruits, berries, leaves, roots and flowers as food. You still need those things, don't you? Of course you do! So you continue to crave them.

Could this not be one source of the blind craving for sweets that seems to drive so many people to overweight? They're hungry! Not for more sweets. They hunger for all the things that come along with the sweet taste in nature, and they're not getting these things in food which has been shorn of everything *except* the sweet taste. So they go on and on, eating and eating, because they are actually starving, they are badly nourished, in terms of the food elements that, in nature, accompany the sweet taste.

How is such a theory going to help us reduce? There's another quite well known scientist who has done a series of startling experiments showing that each of us may inherit quite different needs for various nutrients. Some of us may actually need, to get along well and be comfortable and healthy, twenty or more times of some nutrient than someone else needs. We inherit this tendency, this need.

Dr. Roger J. Williams of the Department of Chemistry, University of Texas, said this about his own work, at a public hearing in Washington, D.C. recently.

"My scientific reputation rests upon (1) discovering pantothenic acid (a B vitamin), (2) doing pioneer investigations on folic acid (another B vitamin) and giving it its name, (3) directing for 23 years the Clayton Foundation Biochemical Institute where more vitamins and their variants were discovered than in any other laboratory in the world, (4) doing pioneer research in the field of biochemical individuality which holds vast promise for human betterment through nutritional means, (5) doing pioneer research on the biochemical aspects of alcoholism."

Dr. Williams has worked with laboratory rats which have been bred for many generations to be as nearly identical as possible. Scientists use animals of this kind in many experiments when they want to eliminate as much as possible any individual differences that might invalidate their findings. Testing rats for variations in their need for certain vitamins, Dr. Williams found that to be healthy, some of them needed twenty times more than their fellows.

Using this knowledge, Dr. Williams and his colleagues were able to manipulate diets and discover all kinds of interesting things about these differences in "need" for various nutrients. They could take away from the diets of all the rats certain vitamins and minerals, then give them a choice of alcoholic beverages or water to drink along with their meals. Some of the rats chose the alcohol. Others were apparently "natural" teetotalers, and never touched the alcohol. Some of the rats eventually became complete alcoholics.

Putting the missing nutrients back into the diet in abundant amounts, these researchers watched the alcoholic rats gradually drink less and less alcohol, until they were drinking nothing but water again. They were cured of alcoholism, by the simple addition of nutrients that they apparently needed in much greater amounts than the rats who were never attracted to the alcohol.

Does it not seem possible that sugar addiction may have the same source? Isn't it possible that the members of a family who have inherited needs for certain nutrients far greater than other members of the same family, may eat and eat until they are grossly obese, because they crave not food exactly, but the nutrients that should be in the food for which they have this excessive need? If, guided by their sweet taste, they are led to sweet foods from which all the nutriment has been removed—things like soft drinks and candy, mostly, they must go on eating or drinking, desperately trying to still the pangs—not of hunger in terms of calories, but craving for desperately needed nutrients.

Dr. Williams' rats were bred to be as nearly identical as possible. If, among animals like these, some may require as much as twenty times more of certain nutrients than others, just consider human beings—especially in a melting-pot country like the United States—where, for generations people have been reproducing to be as varied as possible! We have genes from all corners of the globe, all mixed up in a glorious genetic pool that guarantees that no two Americans will ever be anything at all alike. How do we know that the fellow who eats compulsively until he is tragically overweight is not just suffering from a terrible, excessive need for more vitamins, minerals, whatever, and he's simply not getting it in his food, so he must eat more and more?

Once again, we see what food technologists have done to such a victim. They have removed from the food he eats in excess—sugar and processed cereals—most, if not all, of the nutrients that are in the original food except carbohydrate. The more he eats of these foods, the more hungry he becomes for the missing food elements, doesn't he? Where is he going to get them except in food?

To test this theory, we would obviously have to engage sets of identical twins who have inherited a tendency to overweight. One twin would be fed, from babyhood on, the most nourishing, most natural foods possible. He would satisfy his taste for sweets with fruits and vegetables only, and, in addition, he would be given, throughout life, massive amounts of all the known nutrients such as minerals and vitamins. The other twin would go his own way, eating whatever he wished to eat—"the average American diet," and taking no food supplements. We'd weigh them from time to time. The impossibility of ever conducting such an experiment becomes immediately apparent. Where and how could you interest enough people in becoming subjects of such a study? How could you ever guarantee that they were indeed following the dietary course laid out for them?

Dr. Williams believes that human beings may have as great or greater variation in their nutritional needs than animals. We know that vitamins are intimately involved with the way the body uses food—that is their chief function. Many minerals are known to be associated directly with such metabolic disorders as diabetes—zinc, for instance, which is only now being investigated with great thoroughness, in relation to human needs. The zinc which occurs naturally in sugarcane and cereals is removed almost entirely when these foods are processed into white sugar and refined cereals. Could not lack of just this one mineral be an important cause of metabolic disorders, obesity among them, in persons who eat lots of these two foods and who may, genetically, have much greater than average need for this one mineral?

Who could believe that the presence or absence of a mineral that occurs in such small amounts could be so important? Well, who could have believed, years ago, that the element iodine, in almost microscopic amounts, must be present in foods, or people develop terrible disorders of body and mind! Who could have believed that a kind of anemia that kills could be cured by—once again—almost microscopic amounts of a certain vitamin B12?

Our food technologists are specialists each in his own field. They are not specialists in nutrition. It is their job to present you, the customer, with attractive, well-preserved food that will keep for months on a shelf. It is their job to continue to produce new products, each one farther and farther removed from what the natural food originally was. If any or all nutrients are lost in the process, well, that's too bad. But the food has to meet all the standards of the supermarket shelf, doesn't it? If you insist, we'll shoot a few vitamins into the mix, will that satisfy you? No, it won't— especially not if you're one of the people with excessive requirements for these and the many other nutrients *that are never returned to food after they have been removed.*

Why bring up this whole subject anyway? For a very simple and sound reason. If you are overweight because of a craving for more and more food due to an inherited excessive need for vitamins and minerals, it may help you to reduce, don't you think, if you do everything you can to satisfy that need *with wholly natural food* and, because of your desperate plight, with a food supplement that will provide large amounts of some of those nutrients you may need.

The food part of this is easy to take care of. Just by skipping high carbohydrate foods, you are guaranteeing that you will eat foods in which there are plenty of food elements: meat, poultry, fish, eggs, dairy products, fruits and vegetables. These are the foods in which there are, generally speaking, more protein, vitamins and minerals than any other foods. You have omitted from this list only one essential category of foods: the seed foods—cereals and nuts. But you have also omitted those foods which are all, or nearly all, carbohydrate, shorn of every other nutrient.

The complete food supplement part is not so easy to come by as you might think. We simply don't know about many minerals, for instance—whether they are needed in human nutrition or whether their occurrence in food is an accident, due to soil conditions or contamination. Nor do we know,

112

about many of them, how much is a safe amount to include in a supplement, or in what chemical form they should be taken. On some of the vitamins, we are still turning up new complexes and discovering new combinations in which they exist in foods. How can such things be approximated in a tablet or a capsule?

Do the best you can. There are only two vitamins that present any hazards in overconsumption: vitamin A, which should not be taken in larger doses than 50,000 units a day and vitamin D which has caused trouble when taken in enormous doses. The B vitamins and vitamin C are water soluble, hence any overdose is rapidly eliminated. Individual vitamins should not be taken by themselves unless your doctor is watching for any signs of imbalance. Take a complete supplement, as complete as possible. And take it every day. Don't just plan to take it when you get around to buying it. Make it a regular part of your diet, every day.

The recent nation-wide interest in organically grown food is likely to bring to light other aspects of this matter of individual nutritional requirements and how they can be satisfied with food. Organic food enthusiasts believe their methods of gardening and farming (that is, returning everything to the soil so that the soil is constantly enriched rather than being impoverished) produce food far richer in trace elements and, in many cases, vitamins, than food grown with commercial fertilizers and pesticides.

The Department of Agriculture has made some unconvincing, half-hearted efforts to prove them wrong. But the facts seem to be clear. Soil which is cropped year after year, with nothing returned except the few minerals present in (inexpensive) commercial fertilizer, is bound to be deficient, eventually, in many trace elements which we need for good health.

Chromium, for instance, was recently shown to be intimately involved with the way the body uses carbohydrates. Who ever thought of using chromium for anything other than decorating automobiles? But it has been seriously recommended that we begin to enrich foods with chromium in the hope of preventing blood sugar disorders. Isn't it possible that a large part of our troubles with refined sugars and starches may be that the chromium, along with many other trace elements, is non-existent in the final supermarket product?

And can we not also assume that soil in which chromium is lacking will produce food lacking in chromium? The same is true of the many other trace elements whose peculiar names are just now becoming familiar, like molybdenum and boron. It may be years until our agricultural experts get around to testing soils and the crops grown on them, observing the methods used by individual farmers and the results in nutritional value of foods. Considering the magnitude of the agricultural behemoth that is presently responsible for producing supermarket food, with the whole operation geared to bigness and machinery, this kind of test may never prove to be possible.

Meanwhile, people who raise much of their own food organically, as I do, feel that the infinitely better taste and quality of their carefully grown produce indicates superior nutritional quality as well. The day somebody comes along with a test for chromium, I'll pit my lettuce, beans and tomatoes against commercially grown ones any day! Mine are grown beneath a deep, permanent 20-year mulch which has been slowly breaking down into fine, crumbly top soil for all these years. And I wager there's lots of chromium in that topsoil.

CHAPTER THIRTEEN

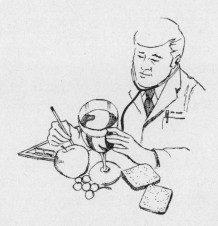

DON'T I HAVE TO ASK MY DOCTOR?

F OR A DOCTOR to prescribe a successful reducing diet, one must assume that he knows a great deal about cooking, modern food and food processing, as well as food preparation at home, the kind of food sold in supermarkets, served in the restaurants or company cafeterias where his patients eat—in addition, of course, to his knowledge about nutrition in general: proteins, carbohydrates, fats, vitamins, how they are used by the body and so forth.

From the medical profession's own publications, one is dismayed to learn that quite the opposite is true. There are not very many medical men pleading for the teaching of more nutrition in medical schools, but the ones who are making any statements at all are saying things that startle and confound.

In 1963 the Council on Foods and Nutrition of the AMA issued a report on *Nutrition Teaching in Medical Schools* in which they expressed concern that maybe doctors were not learning enough at school about the subject. Perhaps, they said, "In each school there should be at least one staff member of professional rank with appropriate training, experience, and a primary interest in nutrition." *One staff member!*

"Students should be taught the basic principles of nutrition as a unit, preferably during the first two years." Instead, it seems that medical students pick up smatterings of information about nutrition in classes in biochemistry and physiology. But the idea that student physicians should devote any time at all to learning the basic facts about what people eat and what they should eat doesn't ever seem to occur to anybody planning medical school curricula. You prescribe a diet to treat a disease. There is apparently no recognition of the fact that eating a good diet throughout one's life may make all the difference between health and illness.

In 1960 the *New York State Journal of Medicine* (October 1), published an article revealing that the average doctor knows almost nothing about nutrition. Said Dr. Richard H. Barnes, "Overemphasis during the vitamin era may have diverted the medical schools and the practicing physician away from learning the fundamentals of nutritional science. Whatever the explanation may be, only a handful of medical schools teach an appreciable amount of nutrition. Physicians frequently must rely completely on the advice of dieticians or consulting nutritionists. They may not be able even to evaluate the adequacy or soundness of this advice. Patients with specific questions regarding their diet are sometimes parried with generalities or perhaps told to read up on the subject in a nutrition book."

Dr. Fredrick Stare of Harvard University wrote in *Nutrition Reviews* a bit earlier that "in many instances very little attention is directed to organization and coordination of nutrition teaching. . . . Nutrition has not yet found a home among the basic medical sciences."

Charles S. Davison, writing in *Science and Food,* a publication of the National Research Council, said, "Nutrition is not an interesting subject to most physicians until they are driven to learn something about it, and most are unable to keep up with the current literature, particularly when it is not directed to the physician in this field. It is just not possible for the physician to keep up with the finer ramifications of this subject . . . The physician is not in a position to know what to believe, or what not to believe, unless it comes from some relatively authoritative source."

Is the situation improving? In June, 1966, the *American Journal of Public Health* published an article by Robert Shank on "Nutrition Education in Schools of Medicine." "Undoubtedly," said he, "there is great variation in the quantity and quality of nutrition information and experience afforded medical students in the 90 different schools of this country. . . . limitation of time and staff experience may prevent consideration of the cultural factors and dietary customs which contribute to the occurrence of these (nutritional) disorders in a population and make modification of the diet difficult."

By 1967 the Federation of American Societies for Experimental Biology published an article which sounds alarming, on the subject of nutrition education in medical schools. Said Dr. J. F. Mueller, "I believe it is fair to say that general dissatisfaction exists among nutritionists in general with the quality of nutrition education in medical schools." He says that there has been no follow-up of the AMA recommendations, made in 1962.

He says, "If one defines nutrition as the science which

117

deals with food, its components and its ecology in human metabolism, then the problem becomes enormous. . . . The medical profession has lagged far behind the biochemists, the agriculturists and home economists in producing highly trained specialists in nutrition . . . I doubt the necessity of a formal course in nutrition although it probably is desirable at some late stage in the training process . . . *If we were successful in interesting one man out of each class in a career in medical nutrition, imagine what an impetus this would be!"*

And in the September, 1968 issue of *Nutrition Today,* Robert H. Barnes, M.D. of the University of Washington, writes on what he calls, "Doctors' Dietary Antics." He says, "Many physicians practice dietetics by the feel of their stomachs. The advice they give their patients about diets and the orders they write in the hospital frequently, no, almost usually, one might say, are based on their own food fancies. When personal tastes fail them, physicians fall back on hearsay or, apparently, resort to poor guesswork."

In a local hospital, Dr. Barnes studied the diet instruction sheets sent to the hospital dietician and questioned some of the doctors in the hospital about what they would prescribe for certain disorders. Far more patients were on special diets than should have been, says Dr. Barnes, almost as if the doctor felt he was not performing his duty if he did not "do something to upset the poor soul's ordinary eating habits." *On an average day, every other patient in the hospital was on some kind of special diet.* At great additional expense, of course.

The terms in which the diets were ordered from the hospital kitchen were, in many cases, totally meaningless. "Ulcer diet" or "semi-soft diet" or "general diabetic diet" are items which no dietician with the best training in the world can understand or follow. One doctor asked the nutritionist for a "cardiac diet" for his patient. When asked what he meant by that he said he didn't quite know what it was, but thought it had something to do with cholesterol. "The gall bladder" diet apparently has something to do with restricting fat. How can the dietician tell, asks Dr. Barnes, whether this ambiguous term means to restrict all fat, or to cut fat by 40 grams a day, or 50, or more? The words "high" and "low" as applied to hospital diets are nearly meaningless. How high? How low? The doctor seldom seems to know and the dietician is left pretty much to her own devices.

Or the dietician is told to serve the patient "Doctor So and So's diet," with no further instructions. Or she is told to give another patient "the American Dietetic Association's 1500 calorie diet—but low in fat." The amount of fat in this diet is 70 grams, says Dr. Barnes. If you decrease this amount, then it is no longer a 1500 calorie diet, and the entire diet must be adjusted to make up the difference.

On a diet described by the doctor as "low salt" or "low sodium," one doctor ordered 250 milligrams of salt, another 5000! Asked what they would recommend as a diet for a patient with a duodenal ulcer, 60 physicians listed six entirely different diets.

For a diabetic patient, one might think there would be some modicum of agreement in the medical profession. Yet five doctors prescribed a total calorie intake of 1000 when asked this question, while others prescribed 1500 calories, and five physicians allowed the patient 2500 calories. As to protein, some doctors thought the patient should have a given amount, while others prescribed twice as much and five doctors said he could eat all the protein he wanted. In limiting carbohydrate (starches and sugars) some doctors said the patient should have no more than 100 grams of

119

carbohydrate daily, some said 150, some 200, others said 225 and one physician allowed this hypothetical diabetic 250 grams of carbohydrate a day! And diabetes is a disorder in which the patient has lost the ability to handle carbohydrate foods successfully!

"No portion of the human body seems to confound physicians more than the gastrointestinal tract," muses Dr. Barnes, "Writing a diet for a patient ailing in this dark and mysterious region seems to fill us with bewilderment." He does not believe that older doctors have any better knowledge of dietetics than younger ones. All suffer from such lack of understanding of the whole matter that he suggests devoting an entire general staff meeting to the subject! He does not explain how doctors can hope to learn all the infinite complexities of nutrition and dietetics in one staff meeting. The hospital he checked is not uncommon, he says. Most hospitals have the same problem.

Says Dr. Barnes, "Medical school deans should review their curricula so that graduates can obtain some working knowledge of dietetics and can become considerably more sensible in this essential and costly part of medical therapy. . . . No patient should ever be denied food unless there is a good medical reason for the denial."

But let's suppose you have found a doctor who is one of the favored few who got in his medical school some kind of grasp of what nutrition is all about. When he tells you "Don't get more than 1500 calories a day" how can you possibly know what to eat, faced, as you are, with the selection of food offered you at the supermarket or in restaurants? You buy chicken pies for dinner. How many calories does each contain? It depends entirely on the ingredients and their proportions.

You go to a party and the hostess offers you a brand new

snack which appears to be mostly air. How can you tell how many calories there are in every mouthful? It depends on the amount of fat and carbohydrate they contain. You discover a new dinner roll at the bakery which your family loves. It's so crunchy! Is this due to a lot of added butter? How many calories?

A diet which tells you what to eat on the basis of calories seems bound to fail, if for no other reason than that you do not have a computer for a brain. But, today, the other important reason is simply that supermarkets are vast labyrinths of almost totally unknown combinations of foods. And there is simply no way to thread your way through them and come out with any definite idea of what you have bought in terms of calories.

Let's consider some items from a calorie list appearing in an excellent book on this kind of diet-planning, *Stay Slim for Life* by Ida Jean Kain and Mildred B. Gibson. One serving of Cream of Asparagus Soup from Campbells contains 70 calories if you dilute the soup with water, 106 if you dilute it with skim milk, 138 if you dilute it with whole milk and presumably a lot more if you dilute it with pure cream, which may have happened in any fancy "gourmet" restaurant where you eat it.

Presumably cream of asparagus soup made by any other company would have a different calorie content. If you are eating this particular soup at home, you are supposed to have the time and the patience to:

1. be sure you buy Campbells brand
2. dilute it according to how many calories you want to come out with. If you want to dilute it with water and your family wants to use milk or cream, how do you solve this dilemma, if you start out with only one can of soup?

3. measure "one serving" which will be seven fluid ounces or 7/8 of a standard measuring cup.

If you are eating out, better skip the cream of asparagus soup, since you will have no way of knowing how it was made or how much is in your bowl.

Take another item: creamed dried beef. The book we are quoting states that one serving (½ cup) contains 205 calories. No mention is made of how this is prepared. The amount of calories would, of course, depend entirely on whether skim milk, whole milk or cream was used, how much butter, beef and flour. The figure of 200–350 calories is given for meat loaf—one slice measuring 4 × 3 × ½ inches (and let's all watch while you do this kind of measuring in a restaurant!). Well, whose meat loaf is it and how did they make it? How many crumbs did they add and how much pork and other fatty meat does it contain? Lots of cooks put sugar in meat dishes believing that they taste better that way.

Do you really think you would dare to eat meat loaf anywhere, no matter how carefully you measured the size of the slice—and be absolutely certain you had eaten only 200–350 calories? And if you are on a 1500-calorie-a-day diet, that flexible 150 calories which is the difference between one meat loaf and another is, after all, one-tenth of everything you are allowed for that entire day, so it assumes quite enormous importance.

One-half cup of rice pudding with raisins will cost you 145 calories. Whose rice pudding? How many raisins? And what if you are served rice pudding without raisins? When you get into the subject of pies, the idea that any calorie list can be a guide to the number of calories in any piece of pie is patently absurd. Magazines and cook books these days contain recipes for literally thousands of kinds of pies and pastries. To have any reasonably accurate notion of how many calories you are eating in any pie, pastry or cake you need a complete laboratory equipped to analyze that particular morsel of food before you eat it.

Even such simple foods as cheese present almost insurmountable obstacles to calorie-counting these days. There are some 400 different kinds of cheese available, many of them imported. What good does a calorie list of cheddar, cream, cottage and swiss cheese do you in this kind of wilderness of cheeses? How do you know whether any given cheese is made with skim milk, whole milk or cream? The calorie difference might be immense! And of course with dishes like lasagna, spaghetti, paella, crab imperial, beef stroganoff, lobster newburg, the calorie content depends solely on the amount of butter, cream, mayonnaise, rice, pasta, olive oil and so on that was used to put this gastronomical triumph together. How do you know? How can you measure?

But still almost every article you read on reducing these days tells you that you must see your doctor and he must give you a "diet list" which will be your guide. How could it be? Even with a computer, how would it be possible for anyone to make up a list which would include every item you might buy at the supermarket, plus every variant you or your friends or some cook book author might dream up, using various combinations of all these foods?

One must assume that *any* diet where you count calories has to be a temporary thing. Obviously you cannot go through all the rest of your life carrying lists of foods about with you, even if these lists contained all the foods which you will encounter on any given day in the supermarket, a restaurant or a friend's house. How can you call this kind of eating "re-educating your eating habits?" I suggest this is one of the main reasons why calorie-counting has gotten us almost nowhere as a reducing plan for a modern individual who must perforce eat what is available in modern society.

There are, of course, people who stay slim counting calories. Through long practice they know about how many calories any dish they are served might contain. They know, in general, how much one serving of soup or crackers, whipped cream or salad dressing will use up of their calorie budget. They know, too, that sugar and fat contain more calories than other foods and they have to be on the lookout for sugar and fat concealed in any food. The computers in their brains must start clicking at this point, or they must consult the calorie list they carry with them.

How do the doctors solve these problems for themselves and their families? A quick glance through several years of medical news journals full of photographs will show you that lots and lots of doctors never solve them, for they are anywhere from 20 to 80 pounds overweight themselves. But the ones who appear to be reasonably slim—what do they eat?

Two writers recently interviewed 87 of the top nutrition authorities in the country and reported in a women's magazine on what they and their families actually eat. These men are, we are told, worried about what is happening to us in a society where food is so plentiful and exercise is something everybody tries to avoid. And most of them are terribly concerned about cholesterol, that fatty substance which, some researchers believe, is responsible for our present high incidence of circulatory disorders—heart and artery troubles. The key words probably, in the thinking of most of these men about food are "avoid cholesterol." Most of them

124

apparently are trying to lose weight or struggling to keep their weight normal.

Here are just a few selected details of how these men, the top nutrition experts, arrange their eating.

One doctor gave up eggs nine years ago, stopped using butter or margarine seven years ago. He now has some 5 or 6 kinds of jam on the table to choose from. We presume he eats this on bread—baker's bread—or else just by the spoonful.

Another doctor who admits, we are told, *that he is addicted to sweets,* eats cereal, toast, marmalade and coffee for breakfast. One can well believe he is addicted to sweets, for this high-carbohydrate breakfast would almost guarantee this. He says he must have a candy bar in late afternoon to get through the day. Dessert at his home is served at nine in the evening. It consists of fruit, pie or ice cream. Before going to bed, he wolfs down an additional melted cheese sandwich. He says that "treats like chocolate layer cake, sweet rolls and eggs are reserved for Sunday."

Another doctor who said little about what he eats during the day admits that he is "liable to eat all through the evening—peanuts and cookies are my weakness."

A former U.S. Surgeon General (that means he was in charge of all public health programs in this country) has never had anything but coffee for breakfast for 25 years. He eats no lunch. He is ravenously hungry for dinner and eats, he says, twice as much for dinner as he used to eat for both lunch and dinner. So now he has cut down on what he eats for dinner!

A professor of physiology whose books on diet are among the most sensible available today keeps a box of almonds and apricots on his bedside table, we suppose to keep from col-

125

lapsing with gnawing hunger during the night. This may be one way to stabilize blood sugar levels, of course, but it seems unlikely that foods containing as much carbohydrate as almonds and apricots would do the trick. (Dried apricots are 85 per cent carbohydrate. Still, they're better than jelly beans or chocolate bars.)

An expert on heart health admits, "I have to struggle all the time. I love to eat." He, too, has practically eliminated eggs and many meats from his meals. The cholesterol, you see!

The man who is most often quoted in general magazines as the expert, par excellence, on anything pertaining to nutrition has cold cereal and a sip of orange juice for breakfast. That's all. Eggs or any kind of breakfast meat are off-limits because they contain cholesterol and other animal fats. These self-imposed restrictions pose the day's touchiest dietary dilemma, according to the article. "What the hell are you going to have (for breakfast)?" this distinguished expert asked the reporter. He settles for mixed dry cereals.

At one restaurant lunch with a group of businessmen, he decided to astound them, because he knew they would watch what he ordered. While the men ordered meat and potatoes, the nutrition expert ordered vichyssoise. Nothing else. This was his entire lunch. His strongest conviction is apparently that one should avoid animal fat, since this is what causes heart attacks, it is said. Why he should then order a luncheon that contains such large amounts of animal fat is a mystery, or perhaps he simply does not know that vichyssoise, in a good restaurant, would consist almost entirely of heavy cream, plus a few potatoes and seasonings. Heavy cream is 37 per cent animal fat. So this expert who would not eat bacon or eggs for breakfast because of their animal fat content has a lunch of almost nothing but animal fat plus a little starch.

Another doctor has eaten no eggs, no cream or milk, no butter for ever so long. He admits that his intake of fat is *dangerously low*. He eats meat only once a day, so it appears that his intake of protein is also dangerously low, unless he is making some kind of heroic effort to get protein in some food other than eggs, meat or dairy products. I wrote and asked him how he gets the recommended 65 grams of protein a day with no eggs and one serving of meat. He did not answer me.

The American Medical Association's official expert on nutrition smokes two and a half packs of cigarettes a day, because he is "hard working and tense." He drinks low calorie soda at coffee break time, believes he should weigh less than he does, but, he says, he does not "intend to deny himself certain cravings."

Far more disturbing are other details that came out in interviews with these, the nation's greatest experts on nutrition and, presumably, normal weight. "Several described their children's eating habits frankly as 'bizarre,' but almost all parents do little but try to keep consumption of soft drinks, candy, chocolate and desserts to reasonable levels."

Their wives cut down on cheese and when they buy cookies for their children "and they often do," they buy "plain ones." Quite a few of the wives were five to ten pounds overweight. "There were a number of overweight children," say the authors, "but none was seriously obese and in almost each case the doctor-father felt that the overweight was a temporary problem of adolescence that the children would outgrow." Famous last words, see chapter 10.

Quite a number of these families get along by fooling themselves about their craving for food. They do not talk about food. Nobody ever compliments the cook on a delicious dish. One couple does everything they can to ignore the food entirely and concentrate on elegant crystal, china and fresh flowers on the table.

"For particularly insistent hunger pangs," say the authors, speaking for other "nutrition experts," "they use such appetite depressants as soup, fruit, water, up to 20 cups of coffee a day and tobacco."

Of sixty-six of these experts who were queried in detail, 36 had cut down on eggs, 38 used less butter, 38 used less bacon and 40 used less whole milk. Although very few of the experts ever had problems with elevated cholesterol levels and *by no means all of them were convinced that cholesterol of itself is a life-shortening poison,* they had managed to eliminate or almost eliminate from their meals such highly nutritious foods as eggs, many meats, whole milk, butter and most cheese.

Four of the experts have nothing but coffee or coffee and juice for breakfast. Many of them eat cold cereal for breakfast, along with toast. One doctor is so hooked on candy that he dares not carry any change in his pocket for he will certainly spend it on candy in the candy machine in the lobby of his office building.

Almost all the others partake of their particular "forbidden fruit" but in moderation, we are told. None of the men eats what the rest of us would call "three square meals a day." Most of them relax over weekends and have "major splurges," by which we suppose they mean that they indulge themselves in all the high-carbohydrate, high-calorie food they want. Then on Monday morning, back on the wagon!

If you believe, after reading these details, that these folks —among the best nutrition authorities we have, according to official titles and occupations—have comfortably and intelligently solved their own personal problems with food and overweight, then follow right along with their exemplary eating habits. Stuff yourself with candy, drink 20 cups of coffee a day, eat no breakfast or lunch, smoke all day, keep an iron grip on yourself and talk about anything but food so that you can manage to refuse a second helping of meat, excuse your children's overweight by saying they'll outgrow it.

Do you believe that these people have found the right answer to maintaining optimum weight in the best, the least painful way? Aren't they doing just what you have been trying to do—cut down on portions of food, skip or nearly skip breakfast and perhaps lunch as well, eliminate fat as far as possible, get your mind off the tormenting thoughts of food which pursue you relentlessly? Well, have these folks worked out any better solution for the problems than you have? Have you managed to reduce and maintain your normal weight this way?

If you have failed, and failed miserably to keep such a schedule, if you find that you just can't get from one meal low in protein and fat to the next without suffering agonies of hunger and faintness, crankiness and cravings, then perhaps another method of reducing is what you should try— the one recommended in this book. Look back at the names and affiliations of those physicians mentioned earlier in this book who are curing obesity with the high-protein diet. They are all professional men, either physicians specializing in treating obesity or related diseases, or they are researchers working on these problems in laboratories.

There seems to be no commercial reason why they should recommend the low-carbohydrate diet unless it works. They are not making any money selling pills, salad oils, diet foods, low calorie sodas, exercise machines, massage machines or any of the other products which are sold regularly to overweight people.

How does it happen that the 87 "top" nutrition experts in the country, most of them apparently concerned about overweight, do not follow the low-carbohydrate diet themselves? Furthermore, why do many of them attack the diet in book reviews or articles read by lay people? I don't know why. For a long time I have been writing letters asking this question of many an editor, physician, writer or nutrition expert who has written pieces in which they attack the whole idea of the low-carbohydrate diet as unscientific, unsound, unsafe, unwise. I have never gotten from any of them any reasonable answer.

Here is a sample. *Good Housekeeping* publishes a reprint of an article entitled, "The Risks of That New Eat-All-You-Want-Diet." The booklet says in part "Basically, this diet drastically limits to 60 grams the amount of carbohydrates (sugars and starches) you can eat daily. But it permits you to eat all the protein and fats (from meats, fish, cheese, dairy products) you want. Most people normally consume from 300 to 400 grams of carbohydrate a day." They quote Dr. C. Glen King, associate director of the Institute of Nutrition Sciences at Columbia University, who says that "a 60-gram carbohydrate diet drives the body to a limit of tolerance." He says several factors in this diet could "place a person at the point of a health risk." Then Dr. King calls the diet "a lot of foolishness."

Dr. Philip White (he's the director of the Food and Nutrition Board of the AMA who, you remember, smokes two and a half packs of cigarettes a day to still the hunger pangs) says that no one should go on this diet without the guidance of a physician. (What kind of a physician, Dr. White? One who might advise smoking two and a half packs of cigarettes a day to cut appetite, or one who might advise drinking 20 cups of coffee a day, as another "expert" does, to keep on going somehow without nourishing food?) Dr. White goes on to say that certain foods which normally contribute essential nutrients such as vitamin C from fruits and calcium from milk would be almost eliminated in a low-carbohydrate diet. He also says there are "no studies which will support that a low-carbohydrate diet will lead to a loss of body weight unless total calories are also controlled."

In every diet recommended in these pages there is ample vitamin C and calcium, especially if one likes cheese. The low-carbohydrate diet, in its bare essence, recommends eliminating from one's meals two kinds of foods and only two kinds of foods: sugar and foods made from refined carbohydrates. Neither of these foods contains any vitamin C or any calcium to speak of.

Dr. White's statement about there being no studies which will support the idea that the low carbohydrate diet will lead to a loss of weight unless total calories are also controlled very cleverly skirts the main idea behind the low-carbohydrate diet as if it did not exist. The idea behind the low carbohydrate diet is precisely that, because of the nature of the diet, *one will not overeat, one's appetite will regulate itself and the whole matter of calories becomes academic.*

Well, I wrote to *Good Housekeeping* and asked them why they stated in this leaflet that "limiting carbohydrate intake to less than 60 grams a day is an unbalanced diet that can possibly promote nutritional deficiencies." I pointed out that the sample low-carbohydrate menus which were listed in *Good Housekeeping* provided plenty of all the required nutrients.

I had a very nice letter from a dietician of the *Good*

Housekeeping Bureau who told me, in part, "although the recommended diet in the article is relatively well balanced, ... the average person would probably not obtain such a good balance. . . . the traditional glass of orange juice, the main source of vitamin C, would probably be omitted because it contains so much carbohydrate. Unless other foods were substituted, this nutrient requirement probably would not be met. . . . it is very difficult to obtain an adequate amount of calcium without drinking milk, another food containing relatively generous amounts of carbohydrate. And finally iron, the nutrient most often missing in the typical American diet, would also probably be limited."

Now consider for a moment what this lady is saying. She is saying that anyone on the low carbohydrate diet will probably not be willing to spend 10 of his 60 carbohydrate grams on orange juice. He might, I believe, wish to make up his vitamin C quota by eating liver at one meal or taking a vitamin C pill. She is saying that milk and other calcium-rich foods are too sharply restricted although one glass of milk contains less than 5 grams of carbohydrate and *one-fourth pound of cheese contains less than three grams of carbohydrate.* You can eat one-fourth pound of cheese every day on the low carbohydrate diet and still have 57 grams of carbohydrate to play around with!

Finally she is saying that a diet which includes unlimited amounts of meat and eggs, shellfish and green leafy vegetables may be deficient in iron! *Heinz Handbook of Nutrition* lists the following foods as those which are the best sources of iron (in decreasing order of excellence) liver, heart, kidney, liver sausage, lean meats, shellfish, egg yolk, dried beans and other legumes, dried fruits, nuts, green leafy vegetables, whole-grain and enriched cereals and cereal products and dark molasses. Of these only the dried beans and fruits, nuts, cereals and molasses would be eliminated or curtailed. And you may eat all you want of the other foods! How would it be possible to lack iron on such a diet?

And is it possible that a typical diet eaten by the nation's 87 "greatest experts on nutrition" is going to be richer in iron than the low carbohydrate diet? Let's see. How much iron is there in a breakfast of coffee, or coffee and juice? Precisely none. How much is there in a breakfast of one bowl of corn flakes, the kind of breakfast eaten by many of the 87 top nutrition experts in the country? *One-third of a milligram of iron!* That's all. The milk eaten with it contains only a trace of iron. And an adult needs 10 to 18 milligrams a day. How much iron would there be in a breakfast of ham and two eggs, the kind of breakfast permitted, nay, encouraged on the low carbohydrate diet? About 6 milligrams. Somehow it just isn't possible to figure out how one would retain a good balance of iron stores on the corn flakes breakfast, but become deficient in iron by eating ham and eggs! If you can figure it out, let me know.

I wrote to Dr. Charles Glen King and asked him what he meant when he said the low-carbohydrate diet drives the body to a limit of tolerance. He answered as follows and we hope you will bear with the medical terminology. Note also the use of the word "marginal." There is a "marginal" risk which I would interpret to mean as an extremely slight risk, wouldn't you?

". . . there is a marginal risk of ketosis when the carbohydrate intake is extremely low in proportion to the combustion of fats and proteins. . . . Normally this is not a problem within short day to day experiences because there is a moderate reserve of glycogen. . . .

". . . for long intervals, the body is put under some physiological stress if the percentage of energy is derived from fats plus the amount of fatty intermediates derived from amino acids. There is a reasonable capacity for adaptation toward extremes, but for general practice there seems to be no need to subject the body to an adaptation process.

"You can find a discussion of this in nearly any advanced standard text in physiology and biochemistry."

I have read such texts and I have read extensively in many medical journals on the subject of the low-carbohydrate diet. Much of what I have read is discussed in this book. I found no mention of any such eventuality in any of the many articles and books I read having to do with a diet in which carbohydrate grams are roughly 60 per day, especially when these are taken in the form of natural foods, not concentrated sugars. So it is difficult to see just how this objection applies.

I wrote to Dr. Philip White of the AMA asking him about his statement and reminding him of Dr. Gordon's experiments with the low carbohydrate diet which were printed in the *Journal of the American Medical Association*. I received no answer from Dr. White.

This is about the percentage and content of replies one expects to get when one writes to inquire about objections to the low carbohydrate diet. This is a land where apparently millions of people eat only one sit-down meal a day— the evening meal, and try to cram all their nutritional needs into that meal, with mountains of high-calorie non-food during the rest of the day. Yet a diet in which all nutritional needs are carefully taken care of in regular two or three hour intervals during the day is railed against as being nutritional foolishness.

The *Good Housekeeping* editor, protesting against the diet, states further that a good reducing diet "should be within the framework of normal eating habits. The goal, of course, is that the eating habits of the dieter can be retrained so that his weight loss is maintained."

What could be more normal eating habits than a diet of meat, eggs, fish, dairy products, fruits, and lots of vegetables of the stem and leaf variety? What is abnormal about it? Is this not exactly the way men ate down through all the ages of evolution up to the time when grains were planted and "civilization" began? What better training could anyone have in these times than training which allows one to eat as much as he wants of such nourishing food, without apology, without guilt, without hunger, without overweight?

On this diet one is trained, you see, to eliminate the nonfoods. These are the foods which are most profitable for the food industry, generally speaking.

The amount of money that can be made selling a cereal which contains, in the words of the AMA booklet, *Let's Talk About Food,* "almost nothing but perfumed air" is very great indeed. And the amount of money to be made selling a new snack food which one is invited to eat all day long is very great indeed. The sugar industry is selling 10,245,000 tons of sugar a year to the American people these days. The candy industry sells three billion pounds of candy a year. Profits in the soft drink industry are astronomical.

It is worthy of note that many of the "top" nutrition experts in the country—those whose opinions are usually sought when any controversy about a new diet arises—have close ties to the giant, wealthy food industry, in many cases to those branches of the food industry which manufacture chiefly high carbohydrate foods.

Dr. Charles Glen King, for example, who was quoted above, was for many years Executive Secretary of the Nutrition Foundation. The Nutrition Foundation, in spite of the ineffably academic sound of its name, is a trade organi-

135

zation of the grocery business. On its Board of Directors are officers of the following companies. We list only a few to give you an idea of just who and what these men are:

The Coca Cola Company, the National Biscuit Company, the Sunshine Biscuit Company, Beech Nut Life Savers, Keebler Company, General Mills, Hershey Chocolate, Quaker Oats, American Can, The American Sugar Company, Pillsbury Company, Standard Brands, plus many more, including an astonishing number of university presidents, heads of foundations and members of government bureaus having to do with food and agriculture.

Dr. Fredrick Stare's department of nutrition at Harvard is housed in a splendid million-dollar building put up for him by General Foods. General Foods does not sell meat, eggs, milk, fish or salad greens. Their specialties are many kinds of cereals, snacks, coffees, desserts, baking ingredients, soft drink mixes, pancake syrup, rice, lemonade and orangeade mix, and chocolate products.

These are the foods of which one could obviously eat very little, on a diet which limits carbohydrates to 60 grams daily. Dr. Stare is also on the board of directors of Continental Can Company which sells bottles in which soft drinks are sold, and so on.

The American Medical Association has an annual income considerably over 20 million dollars. In 1962 they announced that the AMA's biggest source of income continued to be the sale of advertising space in its various publications. The year's total advertising revenue—$9,105,636—represented an increase of almost $200,000 over 1961. Presumably this bounty has continued to increase as years have gone by. It would be possible, but not very interesting, to tabulate how many of these advertising millions come from the food and soft drink industry. The *Journal* of the AMA and several other of its professional publications as well as *Today's Health,* published for the layman, feature usually full-page, full-color, advertisements for soft drinks. The amount of stock in various food and soft drink industries owned by the AMA is a matter about which one can, of course, only speculate.

It's possible that none of these considerations may have the slightest influence on the AMA's official position on reducing diets, or on the position of their official spokesman on nutrition. It would be comforting to think that the AMA speaks on diet with utter objectivity. One cannot help but wonder, leafing through the pages of the journals, just how objective one can be about reducing diets on pages so liberally larded with ads for soft drinks, which, of course, contain not a whit of anything nourishing except for sugar. The ads carry the same message soft drink ads carry everywhere—they refresh you, you come back again and again and again for another bottle; they make a fine luncheon beverage; they stand by you in times of stress or decision-making! All this is suggested very subtly and very effectively, on the pages of AMA publications which, not so long ago, were decorated with ads for cigarettes saying much the same thing. "You'll come back for another." "They get you over times of stress."

There is no way of knowing exactly how other spokesmen on nutrition may be related by strong financial and professional ties to the food industry. Practically all science today exists on research grants. This means relatively huge sums of money given by industry or government to various scientists to carry out certain investigations or projects. Let's say the sugar industry, for instance, wanted to find out

137

more about the relationship of sugar to tooth decay. They might give a financial grant to a qualified scientist to pay for research in his laboratory. A commendable act, one would think. He would then proceed to feed rats or mice certain diets with recorded amounts of sugar. Such experiments might go on for years. At the end, he would report his results and, in his scientific paper, would acknowledge the financial grant he received from such and such a company or industry.

It's possible, certainly, for such a scientist to discover, using money from the sugar industry, that sugar has a very bad effect on teeth and causes extremely serious decay in his laboratory animals. It doesn't seem likely that the sugar industry would be too happy about this, now, does it? So the scientist who would want to receive another grant from the same or a related industry might be hard put to maintain a complete scientific objectivity, for probably no industry will continue to pour money into research which proves that its products are doing people grievous harm.

A friend of ours, overweight for many years, with a family history of diabetes, is a social person who loves to cook. Parties at her house feature tables of pastry, homemade cakes, candy, salted nuts—the works. The refrigerator is crammed with soft drinks. You know the kind of person I mean. Finally, alarmed to find she couldn't get out of her chair one morning—she was stuck fast—she went to her doctor who had long been warning her about her weight. "Cure me," she said, the way most of us do with our doctors. In essence, what she was saying was, "Undo in a month all the damage I've done to myself over the past thirty years." Isn't that what she was saying?

The doctor gave her his special diet #14. It was brief and to the point. Here it is, in its entirety!

OK FATTY
GET TO IT
Eat as much as you want of the following. NOTHING ELSE!!!!! Meat, chicken, fish, eggs, lettuce, string beans, tomatoes, carrots, celery, bouillon, coffee, tea, diet pepsi. No salt. One orange daily. ½ grapefruit daily. If you haven't lost nicely, *you cheated*. Don't cry on my shoulder.

This is a sensible doctor. He has told her, with this diet list, that she never needs to be hungry, that she has a wide range of foods to eat, that she can continue to give and go to parties without boring everybody with her calorie lists. She doesn't have to measure portions. She doesn't have to count calories. She can stuff herself between meals. She can eat a whole chicken if she wants to, every meal. *The point is that, after the first week or so, she won't want to.* Her appetite will have regulated itself. She will, without even being aware of it, be eating a fairly low calorie diet. She will never be hungry. She will not feel deprived or put upon. As she continues to eat this sensible way, she will gradually lose her appetite for sweets. (We wish he hadn't included that diet-pepsi. Maybe today he wouldn't.)

CHAPTER FOURTEEN

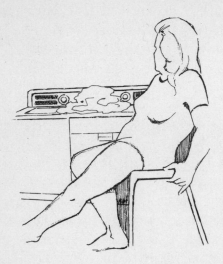

DO I HAVE TO EXERCISE?

I**F YOU WERE** not meant to exercise you would not have muscles. You would exist as a big motionless glob of protoplasm, without arms or legs. You *have* arms and legs. They were meant to be moved. You have a torso which was meant to bend and stretch. Your blood circulation and your heart, your digestion and, most of all, your frame of mind are closely related to how much time you devote to moving around in a healthful, vigorous way.

In this, the last half of the twentieth century every human being, no matter what his weight, should exercise—vigorously, joyfully, enthusiastically, and daily. There is a very good reason for this, which we are sure you don't need to be told. Our lives are becoming increasingly sedentary. No longer do women struggle down to the river's edge, carrying heavy baskets of laundry to beat them on rocks until they are clean. We pop the laundry into the washer and turn on

TV. No longer do we scrub floors, bake bread, pick apples, milk cows or do all the heavy exercising our mothers and grandmothers did. Generally speaking, our breadwinners no longer walk behind plows, pitch hay, wheel wheelbarrows, dig ditches. Perhaps the most significant single change in our way of life is in transportation. Our parents and grandparents walked when they went someplace. We jump in the car, the bus or the taxi. They climbed stairs, we take elevators.

Almost every expert on obesity lists our sedentary way of life as one of the main contributing factors. There are a few who persist in reminding us that to walk off one pound of fat one has to trot 35 miles. And there are still a few doubters who point out that any poundage lost in exercise will be made up as soon as the dieter gets home, because he'll be so hungry and so thirsty that he'll stuff himself.

Sorry, but it just isn't so. Stretch those 35 miles out over 35 days. Walk a mile a day. In a year's time this alone, even with no change in diet, will melt away ten pounds. There's no chance that a walk of one mile every day will render you so ravenously hungry that you'll put the weight back by stuffing yourself as soon as you get home.

On the contrary, it has been carefully proven, many, many times in laboratories that animals which are exercised quite vigorously *eat less by choice than those which remain inactive*. Farmers have always known that to produce fat cattle, geese or any other kind of stock, you pen up the animal and don't let him race around the barnyard. Not only does he store fat because of inactivity, but his appetite increases, apparently due to the inactivity, and he overeats.

With human beings, careful photographic studies have been made of overweight youngsters. They do not move around. On playgrounds they stand and talk. In swimming pools they float and talk. In games they find some way of avoiding exercise.

Here is the story of activity regulating food intake as told in *Science* for April 21, 1967 by Dr. Jean Mayer, one of the world's great authorities on obesity, and Dr. Donald W. Thomas, both of Harvard University. They are talking here of laboratory rats.

"Within the range of moderate activity, rats exercised on a treadmill accurately regulate their energy expenditure and, therefore, their body weight. However, if the activity is too intense, the animals become exhausted, their food intake decreases, and their weight drops. If activity decreases below a threshold level, food intake does not continue to decrease correspondingly. In fact, at very low levels of activity, food intake increases again, a phenomenon interpreted . . . as reflecting decreased glucose (blood sugar) utilization (and exploited by farmers who fatten animals by cooping them up.) Humans respond in a similar manner."

We're back to evolution again. Creatures that were meant to move swiftly and almost continuously (for those are the kind of ancestors we came from) cannot keep their body functions clicking along in perfect trim when they sit all day. Specifically, their appetite mechanism becomes disordered in some way. If they sit around all day, they want to eat more. It's just that simple. So exercise is bound to take off weight in two ways.

First, the extra work burns up more calories. Think of that ten pounds a year loss with no more exertion than walking a mile a day! Secondly, plenty of good, vigorous exercise makes you want to eat less. You don't believe it? Try it and see. And if you find for the first week or so that you do indeed want to eat more when you exercise, then eat more— but eat only the things you will be eating anyway on this diet: high-protein foods, with no more than 60 grams of carbohydrate a day, and no easily assimilable carbohydrates at all. You walk a mile and you're hungry. So you have a piece of meat, a piece of cheese, a hard-cooked egg—that kind of thing. The protein and fat will stay with you long enough that you'll skip that much protein and fat at the next meal. You just won't want it.

There are, of course, hundreds of other reasons to exercise. We don't have to tell you what they are, do we? You have read urgent appeals in your local newspaper and in national magazines by such distinguished men as Dr. Paul Dudley White, to help to prevent heart and artery troubles by exercising. If you are overweight this applies much more directly to you.

There is ample evidence that light exercise after a heavy meal—even a meal which included lots of saturated fat—lowers cholesterol levels in people who tend to have high levels. Shouldn't that fact alone be ample reason for exercising, if there were no other?

There is a wealth of evidence that people who devote their lives to exercising of one kind or another live longer and more healthfully than the rest of us. Ballet dancers probably exercise more regularly and faithfully than anybody else in our society. They live long lives, with good health, brilliant minds and redoubtable spirits up into their eighties and nineties. Have you ever seen a fat ballet dancer?

If exercising makes you eat more so that you will become pathologically fat, why aren't athletes fat? They eat a lot, you may say, but they take it off with the next day's running or jumping, swimming or skiing. So will you. You're not planning any Olympic feats, are you? But you will walk or dance, swim, garden, jog, run, bicycle, climb mountains, or pedal an exercise machine. If you overeat—and we have just assured you that you will not—you'll take it off the next day in the exercise which you are going to continue to do the next day. And the next and the next and the next.

There's another excellent reason for exercising, as you take off pounds. When the pure lard comes off without some exertion you're inclined to be flabby and droopy. Muscles on arms, thighs and especially abdomens have sagged and stretched for so long that they just go on doing it after the fat they enclosed is gone. The right kind of exercise can correct this to such an extent that you can achieve a fine, trim figure at the same time you achieve your optimum weight.

You know this, of course. Everybody knows it. Everybody knows, too, just where to turn for "the right kind of exercise." There are as many kinds of exercise systems as there are people who demonstrate them. All of them are good. The only place they fall down is in the doing.

If there's an exercise expert on TV or radio where you live, turn it on. If it means getting up a half hour earlier, get up. Make all kinds of special efforts at least until you learn the exercises well enough to do them entirely on your own. Then do them. If it helps to exercise in a group, get the family togther, persuade your friends to join you, or neighbors, or your bridge club.

If there is no TV or radio program you can follow, go to your public library and get out a couple of books on exercise. Don't rationalize by telling yourself there may not be such books there. They are there. We guarantee it. Ask the librarian. Or you can inquire at your YM or YWCA. Possibly they have regular exercise programs.

For more extensive exercising, the field is limitless. Join a swimming class and swim summer and winter. Join a hiking club, a folk dance group, a yoga group. If you're the kind of person who has to have a lot of expensive gadgets around to get started at any new activity, then buy something, anything. Get a bicycle, an exercise machine, a pair of skates. Maybe they will reproach you. Maybe you'll feel compelled to use them because you spent all that money!

The amount of money you spent won't take off the pounds, or slim and trim the figure. You have to do that yourself. Don't get a bicycle and then discover you have no place to ride it. Don't buy skates and then find there's no place to skate. The reason walking is usually recommended as the best possible form of exercise is that it is available for anyone. Prisoners in solitary confinement can walk the length of their cells and back. There is no one who cannot arrange somehow to find the proper place to walk if he really wants to walk.

Lately there has been a lot of enthusiasm over what is called jogging. This is fast walking combined with slow running. It's not tiring. It's invigorating and restful. You get a lot of good fresh air. You may meet some nice people who are also jogging. Get a book on jogging and get started, if it sounds interesting to you.

No matter what you decide to do in the way of exercise, get started. Right away. Every day you postpone it means another day lost in the battle, another day for you to be stuck inside this unattractive, bulky, unwieldy and unhealthy frame. Every day you exercise is one day closer toward the goal of good health, good figure, good humor, contentment with your own looks and your own willpower.

CHAPTER FIFTEEN

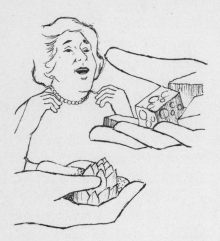

THE MONOTONY OF IT!

THE OTHER DAY I spoke to a friend who had lost 30 pounds on the low-carbohydrate diet and was planning to lose 50 more. She was eminently satisfied. In fact, she had only one complaint. The diet is monotonous, she said. Monotonous? How? Well, she said, there's just nothing to eat but steak, steak, steak, or chops, chops, chops or maybe hamburger and a couple of vegetables. It gets monotonous after a while.

What about eating other cuts of beef in addition to steak, we asked? Well, she had never tried such things as pot roast or flank steak or dried beef or corned beef or any of the other kinds of beef that are just as easily available as steak and hamburger. And just as cheap.

We asked about pork. She had never eaten much pork before she went on the diet. Maybe she could persuade herself to eat some pork from time to time. We asked about

146

lamb and veal. Never occurred to her that she might like them. Poultry? Of course, she ate some roast chicken sometimes. Never tried fixing the chicken some other way than roasting it? And what about turkey, duck, cornish hens, goose?

Did she ever eat fish? Well, no, she never cared much for fish. We pointed out that fish is the least expensive high protein food there is, so one could certainly afford fish at least several times a week.

Was she eating cheese? Yes, but the same old cheese gets monotonous, too, We asked why, then, didn't she try other cheeses than "the same old one?" That seemed like a good idea, she said. We added that there are about 20 different types of cheese, ranging all the way from the hard grating cheeses like Parmesan to soft cottage cheese. Within each of these 20 groups, there are almost endless varieties, including Brie, Edam, Roquefort, Munster, Bel Paese, Cheddar, Swiss, Gruyere, Gouda and so on. Maybe she would. And eggs? You could get mighty tired of fried eggs for breakfast every day, she told me. So why do you fry the eggs every day, I asked. She didn't really know.

We got onto vegetables. It developed that she didn't like eggplant, cucumbers, celery, turnips or squash. She had never tasted artichokes or avocados, didn't know what they were, in fact. Nor had she ever bought any salad greens except iceberg lettuce, which is about the least interesting of them all. So her vegetable list boiled down to several kinds which she ate, fixed in the same way, day after day. Of course it was monotonous!

But the monotony exists only in the mind of this reducer and in the peculiar food habits she developed before she went on the diet. It's not the fault of the diet if the dieter has trained himself carefully from childhood on to enjoy

147

only one or two kinds of meat and three or four kinds of vegetables. The way to settle such a complaint, of course, is simply to widen your horizons and begin to enjoy the fabulous selection of foods the rest of us have been enjoying for years!

It is surprising to find that, in criticisms of the high protein diet, one of the objections is usually "the diet is monotonous." It seems that specialists in food and diet have convinced themselves that one simply cannot plan interesting menus unless he includes every boxed and packaged high-carbohydrate mix that just came out of the kitchen of some big food company.

Many Americans are so loyal to one brand of cereal that they eat it every morning for breakfast, then they have the same soup, sandwich and pie for lunch every day and come home to pizza, steak, hamburger or hot dogs for dinner. Since they are not on a diet, it would never occur to them that such a way of eating is monotonous. But as soon as you restrict any one of these favorite foods—the cereal, the pizza, the apple pie, you have committed a grievous sin by forcing them to eat a monotonous diet! That's what they say, anyway.

I said some of these things to my friend and she agreed half-heartedly that she had been a bit narrow in her choice of food. But the reason, she said, is that she can't follow a diet without recipes. Otherwise the diet is monotonous. What kind of recipes, I asked. Every newspaper and magazine you pick up these days contains recipes. Any recipe is acceptable on the high-protein, low-carbohydrate diet except those which contain a lot of high carbohydrate ingredients—flour, cereal foods and sugar, chiefly, along with such foods as beans, rice, peas and corn.

Well, said my friend, she has a good cookbook—*The Joy*

of Cooking. But of course she couldn't use any of those recipes, could she? We got out her copy of *Joy of Cooking,* which is an old classic cookbook published in 1931 and reprinted frequently ever since.

In the meat recipes, we eliminated only those which depend to some extent on flour for their success, like dumplings. Then we counted. There are 46 recipes for beef, 10 for veal, 14 for lamb and mutton, 22 for pork, 24 for ham, 7 for sausages, 39 for organ meats like liver and kidneys. This is 141 recipes—enough for a different meat for dinner every night for about four months, without once duplicating. There are 30 recipes for poultry and there are 53 recipes for fish dishes. There are 23 recipes for lobster dishes. It would be perfectly possible, using *The Joy of Cooking* as your only source of recipes, to cook a different menu every evening for dinner for an entire year without ever duplicating a meat dish, and stay on the low carbohydrate diet.

True, some of the recipes could not be followed to the letter. But what cook ever does this anyway? When the author of *Joy of Cooking* tells you how to mix flour with water or cornstarch to make gravy, you will of course, omit the flour and serve just the meat juice as gravy. When she tells you to dust a piece of meat with flour before braising it, you can see with your own eyes that the amount of flour remaining on the meat is infinitesimal and will not count in your daily carbohydrate score. When she tells you to top a casserole with crumbs, you will omit the crumbs, dust a little paprika on the top of the casserole and nobody will be any the wiser. You will have saved yourself perhaps one carbohydrate point.

What about stews and pot roasts? You can, of course, continue to make these excellent dishes, using any kind or cut of meat that you choose, except that you will be more careful about the vegetables. If there are folks in your family who are trying to gain weight, or who are perfectly satisfied with their weight, you will continue to drop into the stew or the pot roast potatoes, carrots and onions, if these are the vegetables they like. For yourself, you will add celery, peppers, cauliflower, mushrooms or any of the other vegetables you are allowed to eat. The stew or the pot roast will take on a novel flavor from these added vegetables. You will serve your family with their vegetables and yourself with the ones you are allowed. There is nothing the least bit difficult about such an arrangement.

We have spoken in terms of one cookbook only. Most housewives own several. If there is no cookbook in your house and you don't feel like buying any of the excellent general ones available today, get a cookbook out of the public library and copy down some favorite recipes. Or use the recipes in your daily paper. Just omit the flour or bread, the beans or the bread crumbs, the cereal, the corn, the nuts or any other high-carbohydrate ingredients.

How dull and monotonous are meals likely to be on this plan? Let's plan dinner menus for two weeks. For the main course, you can have beef stroganoff one night, calf liver in wine the next, pork roast the next, creole lamb chops the next, broiled salmon the next, or lobster thermidor, crab salad, sauerkraut and pork, roast lamb, weiner schnitzel, corned beef and cabbage, Swedish meat balls, Hungarian goulash, roast turkey—and so on and on.

For vegetables you can vary those which are allowed by using any of the cook book recipes except those which involve quite large amounts of flour, or crumbs. Cauliflower, for instance, can be boiled, steamed, scalloped, sautéed or served with melted cheese or egg sauce or mushrooms. In other words you could serve cauliflower a different way every evening for a week without exhausting the recipes in *The Joy of Cooking*. And you have some 25 or 30 vegetables to choose from!

Are you going to tell me this will be monotonous eating?

Salads should be eaten twice a day by everybody, no matter what their weight, for there is probably no one food any better for us, for a lot of reasons, than fresh, crisp, raw vegetables of almost any kind we like, doused in any of the excellent salad oils available today and flavored with any selection you prefer of herbs, peppers, vinegars, or other seasonings.

Why do you need a cookbook to tell you how to make salads when the rule is the same for all of them? You make sure the vegetables are well washed, cold, crisp and perfectly dry. Nobody can tell you which vegetables *you* prefer. You are the only person who knows that. If you customarily serve nothing but iceberg lettuce with a piece of canned fruit, then you have every right to feel that such a salad selection is monotonous. But don't blame the high-protein diet for this monotony.

Look over the greens at your supermarket. Take home a different kind every shopping day. Get acquainted with it. You can eat any of them in any quantity, mixed with any other raw vegetables you enjoy or decide to investigate. And heaped with any amount of salad dressing you want. Plus eggs, plus cheese, plus thinly sliced meat or poultry or fish in any quantity, plus all the delightful pickles, olives, capers, mushrooms, avocados and onion rings and anything else you may choose. The possibilities are almost endless.

If you are incapable of dreaming up the ingredients of a good salad, then take to your cookbook. The index of *The Joy of Cooking* offers some 207 salad recipes allowed on your diet, plus some 35 or so salad dressings. You will, of course, skip the lima bean salads, the potato salads and the macaroni salads as well as fruits you won't be eating. And the boiled dressings which are made with cornstarch.

Is this your definition of monotony? *The world is yours when it comes to salads.* You just have to let yourself go! Did you ever think you would ever hear anyone tell you that, on a reducing diet?

Suppose you are the kind of person who doesn't like tossed salads. So eat what the newer cooks call finger salads. The rules are the same. You just don't mix the ingredients and toss them. Radishes, celery, peppers, raw cauliflower flowerets, the raw stalks of broccoli, cucumbers, tomatoes, watercress and any or all the green leafy things can be eaten just as they are. Or you can dip the crisp raw things into a dressing or a dip. Any of the sugar-free dressings will do.

We're now up to dessert on your dinner menu. Dessert should be obviously cheese plus a piece of fruit, if you've left room for that on your daily carbohydrate score. You may have the fruit with whipped cream, custard sauce, gelatin (plain, not the flavored kind) or any other kind of sauce you can dream up which will involve eggs and cream and flavoring, but no sugar.

What about breakfast and lunch? For breakfast you may eat everything anyone else eats except bread, cereals, or foods that contain a lot of flour or sugar. Eggs are the standby of most reducing diets and this one is no exception. Eggs contain the highest form of protein, biologically speaking. That is, the amino acids or building blocks of protein are in a better state of balance, hence more useful, biologically speaking, than are the proteins of any other food. Better than meat, fish, poultry, milk or cheese, or vegetable proteins of any kind.

152

In addition, eggs are a most abundant source of the B vitamins, vitamin A, vitamin E, iron and other essential minerals. Egg yolks contain a lot of cholesterol—that evil word for the substance which is presently believed to be a contributing factor in heart and artery troubles. But cholesterol is a fat. And egg yolks are the richest source of all of a substance known as lecithin which is a well known emulsifier of fats—that is, it breaks up fats into tiny globules so that they disperse throughout any given mixture.

It seems reasonable to assume that the lecithin in egg yolk would do for the fatty substance cholesterol just what it does when you put it into a mayonnaise mixture—break up the fat into tiny bits which won't do any harmful things inside your arteries.

So eggs appear to be the best possible breakfast food for a low-carbohydrate, high-protein diet. They are almost half and half protein and fat with almost no carbohydrate. And what can you do with eggs for breakfast, or any other meal, for that matter? Do you really need recipes?

The Joy of Cooking lists in the index 74 different ways to prepare eggs. That should see you through about two months without ever once eating the same egg dish for breakfast, in case you should decide to eat nothing but eggs for breakfast. On the other hand, a few of these egg dishes contain some bread or flour. Some of them, like curried eggs, may be things that would not appeal to you for breakfast. So let's say you can have a different egg dish for breakfast every day for a month, just using the recipes in *The Joy Of Cooking*. Does that sound monotonous to you?

And of course eggs are only one food you may eat for breakfast. Any meat will do just as well and there is absolutely no reason why you should not have for breakfast a piece of last night's roast beef or broiled ham, if that appeals

153

to you. Some folks like fish for breakfast. Fine. Bacon, ham and sausage are old standbys, all with built-in guarantees that you will not eat too much of them. They're too fatty. What about hamburgers? What's wrong with them for breakfast? Nothing. Just skip the rolls or the buns and eat as much of the meat as you want, within reason. Pizza obviously doesn't qualify as recommended food for breakfast or any other meal, since one serving contains about 30 grams of carbohydrate.

What about between-meal snacks? There's nothing to prevent you from eating these all day long if you feel like it, provided of course that you stick to the recommended foods or that you are careful to count between-meal snacks as part of your total carbohydrate count. Does this mean you can blow the whole day's carbohydrate count on one chocolate sundae or candy bar? Of course not. High-carbohydrate treats unbalance your blood sugar levels which you are trying, by means of this diet, to stabilize. Of course you will avoid them. And it will get you nowhere to "cheat a little"—just a few extra points today and a few extra points next week. *The diet won't work that way.*

There's another angle to the problem of what to do about desserts and sugary snack foods. A great deal of scientific evidence points straight to the conclusion that sugar—plain, unbuffered sugar as it exists in soft drinks, candy and many desserts has the physiological aspects of a drug. You can't get along without it, you think, because you are addicted to it, in much the same way that people get addicted to other drugs. You have "withdrawal symptoms" when you try to go without your afternoon coke or candy bar. You get nervous, jittery, depressed. You have butterflies in your stomach. These are withdrawal symptoms and you get over them just as you would get over the withdrawal symptoms of any other kind of addiction—by staying away from that particular drug.

You will not believe it now, but the day will come when you will not want that afternoon soft drink or candy bar. Really. The day will come when you will pass by sundaes and cake, desserts and cookies without a single twinge. You will find yourself avoiding candy stores because the smell of all that concentrated sugar will be quite distasteful to you. Then you will know that you are cured of your addiction.

Perhaps you are already the kind of person Dr. Cleave talks about who likes foods plain without any fancy puttering around with sauces, flavorings and what-not. You like plain broiled meat or fish, plain roast chicken, vegetables with no dressing but butter or salad oil, fruits raw and unadorned.

If you are this kind of person, chances are good that you are not very overweight, for this kind of eating does not by itself generally produce overweight. It's an honest kind of eating. You are hungry for a piece of meat and that's what you eat—not a conglomerate mishmash doused in gravy and spread over a plateful of noodles. You are hungry for an apple and you eat an apple—just that. Not a piece of apple pie, not an apple tart, not an apple dumpling, not a dish of applesauce, but a plain, raw apple. You don't put on much excessive weight eating this way.

But if you live in a family where this kind of eating is encouraged, *along* with misplaced devotion to all kinds of starchy and sugary dishes "because you must have sugar for energy" or because mother was such a good cook, or simply because all such foods are so cheap and so attractive at the supermarket, then you have the same problem other overweight people have. You must get over the deception that you have been practicing on yourself.

155

There is no such thing as being *naturally* hungry for a piece of chocolate cake, because down through the ages that human beings have been evolving, chocolate cake was not growing on trees or bushes. So taste buds have no inherited method of dealing with foods like this. There is no appestat mechanism to tell you when you have had enough. You'll just have to believe me when I promise you that, after you have been pursuing a high-protein, low-carbohydrate diet for long enough to take off the weight you want to lose, you just won't want foods like this any more. You'll find yourself asking for grapefruit or a piece of cheese for dessert *because that's what you really want,* not because you're forcing yourself to observe a carefully controlled diet.

So what are you going to do about other "recipes"— those magic things that somehow take all the terrible monotony out of everyday living? This concept, it seems to me, springs from a notion that it's not really possible to eat a high protein food without, somehow, mixing it up with a high-carbohydrate food in a one-dish meal that is somehow supposed to be more appealing than the high protein food alone. We eat meat balls *with* spaghetti, goulash *with* noodles, sauerbraten *with* dumplings, roast beef *with* browned potatoes, and so on.

There doesn't seem to be any good, culinary reason for such practices, or any good health reason, so long as food is plentiful. There seems to be ample historical evidence that the high-carbohydrate part of our meals was assembled by housewives into attractive and appetizing dishes because there just wasn't enough of the high-protein foods to go around. So you pieced it out with noodles, rice, potatoes, pasta, corn meal, because these foods have always been the cheapest foods.

So think of your high protein diet in terms of gourmet

meals. You're eating expensively when you cut down on carbohydrate. But, actually, in terms of everyday living in modern America, it's perfectly possible to pay almost as little for this kind of diet as you used to pay for the diet which made you fat. And think of the money you'll save in buying clothes, in doctor's bills, in all kinds of special things you must do and buy so long as you are overweight.

To get back to recipes, in case you feel you want to talk more about them. Sit down and make out a list of the food you might have eaten this week, cooking the old way. How many of the recipes can you change by removing the starchy part? Most of them, undoubtedly. Like this. If you serve your family spaghetti and meat balls, eat just the meat balls and the sauce, yourself, along with an enormous salad and all the antipasto you want. If you serve your family roast beef and mashed potatoes, with gravy, add a low carbohydrate vegetable, which you will eat along with as much meat as you want and an enormous salad with plenty of salad oil. You get the idea, I'm sure.

What do you do when you are eating out? In a restaurant the ordering is easy. Skip most of the before-meal treats—no soup, no juice. Meat, fish, or poultry in any amount as a main course, plus one or two vegetables from the low carbohydrate list. After a day or two on your diet, you'll know these by heart and will automatically pick them out on any menu. Cabbage, in slaw or pickled, is a good choice. Along with, of course, salad—as much as you can hold, with plenty of salad dressing. Skip the dessert with a gracious shake of your head and use no sugar in your coffee or tea.

Lunch in a restaurant is a little more difficult if you're eating on a budget. But almost any restaurant serves tuna, ham, crab or salmon salad or sandwiches. If you're not very hungry—and I promise you this will occur surprisingly often—order the sandwich, scrape off the fish or meat and discard the bread. You can do the same with any meat or cheese sandwich. Any egg dishes are acceptable, but lay aside the bread or rolls that come with them. Dessert is off limits, unless you want to spend several carbohydrate units on a half grapefruit, an orange or a piece of melon.

You're invited out to dinner. Your hostess is one of your town's noted cooks. If you know her well enough, explain before you go what foods you can and cannot eat and ask her pardon for avoiding these dishes, no matter how carefully she has prepared them. If she's not that good a friend, you'll have to fake your way through the meal, trying to be as unobtrusive as possible. If the potatoes or the lima beans are served to you, leave them on your plate, well stirred around, so that nobody can tell whether you have actually eaten any of them or not. Eat lots of the meat, seafood or poultry, or whatever your hostess has prepared as her main triumph. Praise it unreservedly. Ask for seconds, if that's the kind of dinner it is.

If the main dish is a real trap like spaghetti, lasagna or paella, do the best you can to avoid the starchy part of the main dish. Concentrate on the vegetables and the salad. Skip the relishes, the rolls, the jams, the fruit juices. When dessert appears—it may be your hostess' favorite chocolate mousse on which you know she must have spent half a day. Ask for a very small portion "because everything was so delicious that I just can't eat much dessert," or something like that. Whether the serving of high carbohydrate dessert you get is small or large, toy with it. Push it around on your plate. You may even eat a small bite of it, if you're sure you won't be tempted to go on and eat the rest. No one will notice that you haven't really eaten any of it.

What about a cocktail party? Usually there are ample

tidbits you can eat in quantity, like cheese, cold cuts, olives, pickles and so on. If you're sure this is the kind of party where the emphasis will be on heavy drinking and heavy eating at dinner, with sparse fare at the pre-dinner round of drinks, better have something substantial before you go. That's not so hard, really—a dish of cottage cheese or a big chunk of harder cheese, a hard-boiled egg or a piece of meat. There are people who believe that one reason for our massive problem of overweight is the elongated time many of us spend on drinks before dinner. Blood sugar levels must sink to abysmal lows in these circumstances, liquor sloshes around inside unaccompanied by any solid food and we arrive at the dinner table so tired and so lit that we don't even know what we're eating most of the time, no matter how much gourmet care has gone into the preparation. And we wolf down much larger quantities than we should have.

A party of this kind can wreak havoc with the best intentions of the most steadfast dieter. You simply go without food for too long a time. Eating some high protein food before you go is the only sensible way to cope with the elongated cocktail party. It's probably not a good idea at all ever to attend a cocktail party which is just that—cocktails —with nothing to tide you over beyond the end of the drinking. Don't go, unless it's near enough at hand for you to nip back home for dinner immediately, or walk to some nearby restaurant for some real food.

What do you do at the PTA meeting or the church social or the neighborhood gathering where six kinds of cake are served along with the coffee? You carefully take a serving of the cake, or cookies, or brownies, or pie, or ice cream, or whatever high carbohydrate dish is offered and you balance it in your hand along with your coffee or tea. You drink the beverage, without sugar. *You do not eat the food.* You

159

slice it up a bit, shove it around on your plate, while you are busy talking and circulating. No one is ever going to see how much of it you really ate.

We have assumed somehow throughout this chapter that the person interested in reducing with the high protein diet is also the person who plans meals. This is not of course always the case. What do you do if you are served your meals by a devoted mother, wife, sister, daughter, aunt or even maid who loves to keep you fat because, she thinks that's a sure sign you're healthy? And, into the bargain, she loves to cook, and her idea of good cooking, like most peoples', is to heap high the starchy and sugary goodies, while you belch and sigh, then flee to the sofa to collapse after dinner.

You have to make up the rules for your own circumstances. I can't do that for you. It seems most reasonable to ask the cook of the family to read this book and cooperate, for any reason that you feel may be most effective in your case. Health? It may be health, comfort, appearance, you may have to reduce to get a new job, or to have an operation. You may be able to persuade the family cook if she's overweight, to eat as you want to eat, so that she will have to prepare only one meal and never make special dishes for you. That is, of course, the ideal way to do it.

If your family cook happens to be thin, persuade her, if you can, that the high protein diet is the best possible way for her to regulate her weight, as well, without putting on a lot of flabby fat she won't want.

What do you do if you get nowhere with any of these suggestions, if you are told flatly that such an idea is nonsense, that pasta and pie are the best foods there are in the world and nobody is going to eliminate them for your sake just because you read this crazy book?

160

Again you're going to have to solve this your own way. I can only make some suggestions. Arrange to eat more meals out where you can choose your own menu. Leave for work early enough to eat in the same restaurant every morning and let the chef know what your problems are. Chances are he'll be glad to cooperate. If you have to, tell him it's doctor's orders. Sometimes this will work when nothing else does.

If you must carry lunch, lay down the law as to what it shall be. At dinner, eat only the high protein part of the meal, plus whatever vegetables you are allowed and just leave the rest on your plate. No good cook worth her salt will persist in seeing her delicious food rejected meal after meal. She'll change. She'll begin to serve what you want her to serve.

If the protein part of meals is still too scanty, bring home your own cheese and cold cuts. Have snacks during the evening. No beer, no pizza, no soft drinks, no pretzels. Stick strictly to high protein snacks. Have a glass of milk or buttermilk. She'll come round. You'll see. As soon as you begin to have your clothes taken in, your posture and your frame of mind will improve, your head is clearer. You don't fall asleep or want to fall asleep after dinner.

There are individuals with other problems. You may be one of them. Let's say you have been placed on a diet by your doctor which eliminates some of the mainstays of the high protein diet—salads, for example. You're not allowed to eat any raw vegetables, let's say. Tell your doctor that you would like to go on the high-protein diet and ask for his recommendations. Chances are he will be agreeable and you can proceed with the diet, except that you will cook vegetables instead of eating them raw. All other restrictions on your diet can be observed, as usual, except that you will eliminate high carbohydrate foods to keep the carbohydrate content of your diet within the specified count.

If you have allergies to some of the foods recommended on the high protein diet, these, of course, must be eliminated. You are already eliminating them and have learned to live without them. Other diets prescribed for various conditions will have to be considered carefully with the doctor who prescribed them, to see whether they can be fitted into this schedule. It seems unlikely that any doctor is going to forbid you to eat the high-protein, low carbohydrate diet if you are careful to explain to him that you will be omitting all desserts, sweets, candy, soft drinks and so on, because in his heart he knows that this is really the best diet to follow.

CHAPTER SIXTEEN

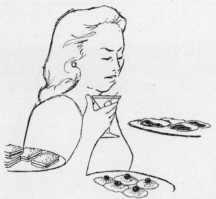

HOW ABOUT A MARTINI?

T HE LOW carbohydrate diet has become famous in part because two California men wrote a book calling this diet *The Drinking Man's Diet*. In this book they recommend eating less than 60 grams of carbohydrate a day and drinking a reasonable amount of liquor, if that's the way you are accustomed to living. In some reviews of the book by an unfriendly press, one would think that its authors were proposing that their readers force themselves to drink whether they want to or not!

The general idea is that alcohol is not used by the body in quite the same way other carbohydrate foods are. So, if you want to, you can use up a few carbohydrate units every day with a cocktail or a glass of wine. A three-ounce martini contains only a trace of carbohydrate, the same with distilled liquors like whisky, gin, vodka and so forth. Liqueurs and sweet wines may have from 2 to 7 carbohydrate units.

163

Beer—18 units in 12 ounces. Club Soda and low calorie soft drinks contain no carbohydrate. One cup (eight ounces) of ginger ale contains 16 carbohydrate units, a cola drink 20. So a highball or two of whisky and water are permissible with no counting. When you get into mixed drinks the "mix" part of the drink is likely to mount up. An old-fashioned counts 4 carbohydrate units, a Manhattan 7, and so on.

Obviously, if you don't drink or seldom drink there is no reason to begin now just because some drinking happens to be permitted on this low carbohydrate diet. On the other hand, if you have avoided going on any diet just because you feel you can't give up your cocktail before dinner, then take heart. You don't have to.

If you are a person who has consistently skipped breakfast, slighted lunch and then had three quick and enormous ones before dinner, chances are you will find on this diet, that you don't need the three quick ones, or, if you still want them, you can space them out over a lengthy cocktail hour and the dinner you eat will no longer be all that enormous. You just won't want so much to eat as you have in the past. If you are used to drinking a little wine with meals, you can still drink wine, but don't for goodness sake take it up just because you're on a diet that allows it!

It's the mixed delights, as always, that will do you in. As soon as you see the hostess approaching with a tray of something rolled in pastry, or sandwiched in crackers, or heaped on slabs of toast, excuse yourself and saunter over to the table where the radishes and celery are laid out.

For your own cocktail parties, taking for granted that many of your friends are dieting in one way or another, it's only generous and helpful to provide them with plenty of rabbit food to keep them munching while the cocktails last.

164

Your own ingenuity is the key. Be lavish with radishes and celery, slice the stems of raw broccoli, and serve them with garlic salt. Put out huge bowls of watercress and other greens with a thin salad "dip" for coating the greens. Tiny raw nubbins of cauliflower head, thin-sliced carrots, pickles, olives, cheese dips—all these things are permitted and inexpensive. Skip the pastries and the crackers, the pretzels, the crispy snack foods which are nothing much but flavored air, salt and starch.

And don't, of course, overdo the drinking. Maybe you've been drinking too much heretofore, so that you could cut your appetite at the dinner table. You don't need to do that any more, remember? You're allowed to eat as much as you want of most of the foods that will be served, remember?

So when you plan your own dinner parties, keep the cocktail hour short. Anybody who must have more liquor can drink it during dinner or after dinner. And those folks who came to taste and enjoy your delicious food will be able to do just that and keep their slim figures as well.

CHAPTER SEVENTEEN

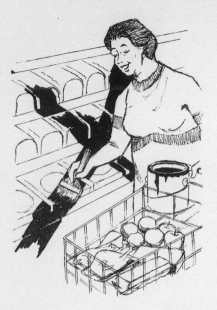

WHAT'S IT GOING TO COST?

Wʜᴀᴛ's ɪᴛ going to cost? You're going to eliminate most of the fairly inexpensive high-carbohydrate foods and you're going to eat the fairly expensive high-protein ones. There's no doubt of it. High protein food is more expensive. This is one reason why high protein foods are so watered down in most menus with high carbohydrate foods. Meat balls are more expensive than spaghetti, so you serve them both. Pot roast is lots more expensive than noodles, so you serve the noodles along with it, to help fill people up.

On the other hand, think of the saving—the things you will just never buy again! Walk into the supermarket and go down each aisle. You will be astonished to find that the counters where you buy meat, fish, poultry, dairy products, fruits and vegetables take up so little room compared to the aisles and aisles and aisles of foods which you are going to avoid.

There's a whole aisle devoted to cookies. There's one whole section of nothing but baked goods—cakes, pies, pastries, rolls, crackers. A big part of the frozen food section is devoted to frozen desserts. You'll walk past that without a sideways glance. These things cost money too, remember. There are shelves and shelves of jelly and jams. You won't be needing those.

The candy section grows larger every year. Cross it off your grocery list. Avert your eyes. Pass by the packaged dessert section without a glance—all those attractive nuggets of sweet, sweet concoctions, made ever so much more sweet and attractive and fruitier than fruit with ever-so-clever chemicals that mimic the taste of the actual fruit. There are hundreds of these chemicals used lavishly in prepared gelatin desserts, in candies, in soft drinks, in processed goodies of all kinds. Just think of all the money you'll save on soft drinks! They are nothing but water, you know, with a rather large bit of sugar and a dollop of dyes and chemicals to make them taste and look like something agreeable.

So now you're past most of the things in the supermarket which you don't intend to buy. You're at the meat counter. Beef, pork and lamb are relatively high-priced, most cuts, that is. But there are plenty of cheaper cuts which are just as nutritious and can be made just as tasty and tender. Poultry and fish are the two least expensive high protein foods you can buy. They are also probably the best high protein foods you can eat, according to information we have from nutrition experts at present, since they contain far more of the beneficial unsaturated fats and less of the saturated fats than do beef and pork, veal and lamb. We've been told by many top men in the field of nutrition, heart and circulatory disorders and overweight that we should eat less

167

of the foods whose fat becomes solid at room temperature—beef, lamb, butter, lard and so on—and more of those foods whose fat is much less solid at room temperature—poultry and fish, chiefly, along with salad oils. So buy your fill of poultry and fish. On one reducing and heart saving diet called the Prudent Diet in which a large number of men were tested for a period of several years, one requirement was that they eat fish and poultry often. Here are some of the rules of that diet in regard to meat:

eat seafood at least 4 or 5 times a week for breakfast, lunch or dinner

eat poultry often, especially the white meat which is low in fat

eat veal frequently, since this is quite lean

eat beef, pork and lamb no oftener than three or four times a week.

There are hundreds of different kinds of fish available almost anywhere these days. You can buy them fresh, frozen, canned, salted, dried. They are excellent protein food, preferable to meat for several reasons that have nothing to do with unsaturated fats. They contain iodine, an essential mineral which is likely to be missing from foods raised inland, as well as many other minerals. They are, generally speaking, much less likely to be doused with the hundred and one chemicals that may be involved with any piece of meat or poultry you can buy anywhere these days. After all, they come right out of the ocean to you, or to the freezing locker or the canning station where the aim is to get them processed as quickly as possible, to save profits.

Finally, from the point of view of the dieter, fish are foods that, somehow, lend themselves well to the kind of cookery that doesn't involve great blobs of carbohydrate additives. Somehow you don't think of fish pie or fish gravy, or fish strewn all over noodles or macaroni or baked into pastry or stuffed with bread. Fish is a delicate, fine-tasting morsel of food that goes somehow very well into the broiler with a dusting of paprika and a little butter and served with nothing much else, save a whopping big tossed salad plus a low carbohydrate vegetable. So if you decide to follow this advice on fish—and it's certainly excellent advice—your meat bills may turn out to be lower than they have been for years. Let's move on to the dairy counter.

Advocates of the diet high in unsaturated fats believe you should use only skim milk products, not whole milk. This means sticking mostly to cottage and pot cheese, with skim milk for other drinking and cooking needs. Cottage cheese is inexpensive. It's an old time stand-by of all dieters.

Butter and milk? What are you going to be needing so much butter for, now that you won't be eating any more pancakes, waffles, cakes, pies, cookies, and all the other things that you have used butter for in the past?

Milk is far more expensive than it should be. So is cheese. But for the amount of nutritive value you get from it, there is little reason to complain. Sure, use powdered skim milk if you like. It's very inexpensive and loaded with protein, vitamins and calcium. Use it to enrich any "recipe" foods you make, like creamed things (you just have to count a smidgeon of carbohydrate here for the flour and the milk you use).

Cream is expensive, too. And you're going to be very pleasantly surprised at how unappreciative of cream you become after a while. At the moment it probably seems that the license to have as much cream as you want with every meal sounds heavenly. What are you going to use it on?

You can't just drink it by the glass, you know. It cloys very soon. It satiates. It nauseates. It's possible that men would be better off if they had never discovered how to separate concentrated cream from milk, for, in the concepts of Dr. Cleave and Dr. Yudkin, cream is not actually a natural food that mankind has had access to down through the ages of evolution. And, let's face it, cream contains lots of those saturated fats which the heart specialists are warning us against. So going very easy on cream would seem to be wise. You'll find it's not hard at all, after a while.

Eggs are the other standby among high protein foods. The experts who place such emphasis on the dangers of saturated fats think possibly you should avoid egg yolk. It's high in saturated fat and also cholesterol, which, we have been told, tends to cause heart and circulatory ills if it's taken in abundance. There seem to be many reasons for doubting the validity of this claim where eggs are concerned. The chick lives on the egg until it's hatched. So far as we can discover whole eggs contain every nutrient needed by chicks and by human beings as well, with the exception of vitamin C. No more "natural" food could be imagined than the egg, relatively safe, inside its shell, from any depredations and meddling by human "technologists" who always somehow seem to think they can develop something a lot better than nature has developed. Men have been eating eggs for hundreds of thousands of years and animals ate them for millions of years before that—all they could get. True, most animals and most men in past ages have not been able to find as many eggs to eat as we can eat today. They had to hunt for their eggs in the nests of wild birds.

Today eggs are produced mostly by hens cooped in huge buildings, who do nothing but lay eggs all day—and sometimes all night as well. There is nothing "natural" about

170

such a formula. Birds of all kinds "naturally" fly, peck at food on the ground, rest, move about and conduct their rather intricate social affairs. What effect modern ways of producing eggs may have on the nutritional content of the eggs is just not known and probably never will be known. After all, there is no way to find out what was the nutritional content of eggs produced a hundred years ago by hens which were allowed to range free and to lay eggs whenever they felt like it—fertile eggs, too, for there was always a rooster somewhere about.

Organic poultrymen still produce their eggs and poultry the old-fashioned way. Their hens still run freely in the open. Most organic eggs are also fertile. There's a rooster in the poultry yard. Their feed is free from hormones and antibiotics. Whether these expensive precautions produce an egg which is far superior in nutritional value and in the quality of its lecithin content is a matter which will be determined in time. Meanwhile, there's at least one world-famous gourmet cook, Roy DeGroot, who displayed on the Today Show two of his own soufflés, one of them flat and sodden, the other (made from organic eggs) high, fluffy and delectable.

Was there perhaps less cholesterol in eggs thus produced? We don't know. We do have some pretty convincing evidence that the kind of fat we are producing in beef cattle that are raised in close confinement is different from the fat of wild cattle that roam about. So possibly eggs do contain more cholesterol than a sedentary person should eat. But you're not planning to be sedentary, are you? Besides this, eggs contain a wealth of other food elements that, it seems quite possible, may counteract any damage their cholesterol may do you. Lecithin, for instance, is more abundant in eggs than in any other food. Lecithin is the world's greatest emulsifier. It breaks up globules of fatty substances into tiny little specks. The egg in mayonnaise breaks up the large amount of salad oil you use to make it, so that the tiny drops of oil are held in suspension and you are hardly aware that you are eating fat. Could not the lecithin of eggs perform this same function inside the blood vessels where cholesterol is supposedly piling up, clogging blood vessels and causing hardening of the arteries?

Quite apart from its lecithin content, the egg contains so much more that is valuable in human nutrition that the idea of cutting down on eggs seems the height of folly in a nation that spends three billion dollars a year on soft drinks, almost seven billion on cigarettes, 14 billion on alcohol. Besides, since you will not be eating cakes, custards, puddings, mousses and other desserts in which eggs play a prominent part, you may find yourself actually eating fewer eggs than you did before.

Aside from high protein foods, you are going to eat vegetables and fruits, aren't you? The vegetables will be quite inexpensive, whether you buy them fresh, frozen or canned. Salad vegetables and the crisp things you will be eating raw whenever you feel hungry are not very expensive. You can usually get just as good fresh produce and canned and frozen things at the least expensive store in town as you get at the most expensive.

Fruits are expensive, but not nearly so expensive if you buy them in season. Sure, the fresh strawberries look ambrosial in February. But they cost an arm and a leg and, after you get them home, you find they don't really taste very good after all, for they've been so long in transit from wherever they were grown.

If you live where you can get out into the country, you can make arrangements with orchard and farm people for apples, melons, pears, peaches, apricots and other fruits in season for far less than you would spend at the supermarket. And the fruit will be ever so much fresher and better. You can save very sizable amounts of money by freezing such foods in quantity, when they are in season.

Raising your own vegetables is, of course, the very best way to economize. You can cram a splendid garden of tomatoes, lettuce, cucumbers, squash, radishes, celery, snap beans and peppers into a small backyard, mulch it to keep down weeds and add to the soil's fertility, use only those organic fertilizers like bone meal, dried manure, cottonseed meal and so on. All these are low carbohydrate vegetables. You grow enough for your entire family for the few pennies you spend for a package of seed or a flat of seedlings. And you get the fine, vigorous, satisfying outdoor exercise of gardening, as an added bonus.

CHAPTER EIGHTEEN

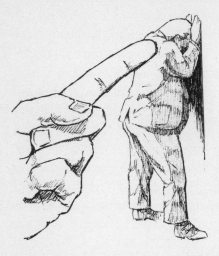

PINNING THE POUNDAGE ON THE QUIRK

T HE PSYCHOLOGICAL mystique that has recently grown up around obesity and overweight is astonishing. Almost anything the sociologists and psychologists can get their teeth into these days degenerates eventually into a situation where these pundits stand aghast at what the common man has managed to do to himself in the past fifty or so years. That he is wholly to blame for his present condition is the usually accepted premise. And explaining the reasons for overweight is no exception.

You're overweight because you love and/or hate some member of your family. You're overweight because you are insecure. You're overweight because you have a deep-seated need for oral satisfaction, because you're afraid of being unpopular, because you feel guilty about something or don't feel guilty about something you should feel guilty about.

You're overweight because you have anxieties and

174

stresses. You're overweight because you like to bite things, chew things, as an act of aggression. You're aggressive—of course you are! Look at the crime statistics! Read Konrad Lorenz! You're overweight because it isn't socially permissible for an adult to suck his thumb. You're overweight because you feel uneasy at social gatherings, because you're easily depressed, because you cannot adjust to life's circumstances, because you work under a great deal of tension, because you feel compulsive about food. The list is almost endless.

No matter what the psychological quirk, if you have it and have some unwanted pounds at the same time, the professional delvers into the slimy depths of personality can usually pin the poundage on the quirk. It apparently never occurs to anybody that the same things which made you nervous and insecure, tense and guilty might be the same things that made you fat! The kind of food you've been eating, for instance.

Medical and scientific journals these days carry an alarming quota of articles on the psychological reasons why people are fat—not one of them alluding to the real reason.

A nutrition expert from Cornell University decided recently that some people are better off fat. If it appears that they are not going to succeed in reducing and that there may be some undesirable consequences if they try, then by all means let them stay fat. A doctor writing in *GP* announces that obesity is a lifelong disease that can only be controlled, never cured. An individual with obesity is a lifelong cripple, he says. If there is an indication that psychological reasons are involved, he should be given psycho-therapy. (Of course people have been saying this about alcoholism for years, but there is quite a body of sound evidence that alcoholism can be controlled by diet and blood sugar regulation.)

Another researcher announces that if all the pleasurable aspects of eating are taken away, obese people will not over-eat. He fed fat people a tasteless liquid diet through a tube and they never took more than 250 calories a day or 500 to 700 calories if they were permitted to watch TV while they ate!

A physician hypnotist told physicians and dentists at a meeting of the American Institute of Hypnosis that dieting is the worst thing fat people can do. They become obsessed with the subject of food, said he, and they are goaded into wanting to eat. "Trying not to eat is like trying not to think of an elephant. The mind is immediately obsessed with the picture of an elephant."

A Danish physician believes that the person who refuses to lose an extra ten pounds does so because he actually needs the fat to keep warm! A Southern doctor, listing obesity as an incurable disease for which the primary cause has not been found, suggests that it provides a real challenge for the physician to "make maximum use of the art and the science of medicine." A New York city nutritionist says that many overweight women who stay at home with their children have few inner resources. They are bored and disenchanted and eat to add pleasure to their lives. No one ever asks *what* they eat when they are bored and disenchanted.

No one in this entire professional group, apparently, has ever heard of the Masai or any of the other nations which live in certain parts of Africa, all of whom are tall and thin, beautifully built, spare, lean, magnificent. They live on diets consisting almost entirely of blood, meat and milk. Carbohydrate foods are all but unknown to them. Is it possible that not a single individual in all these nations that we tend to categorize as "backward" has ever suffered from boredom, anxiety, self-consciousness, timidity or the need to put something into his mouth? If indeed these are the things that make people overeat to the point of obesity, how does it happen that none of these Africans ever overeats to that point?

A New York nutrition expert states categorically that a typical overweight young woman, living in the throbbing heart of one of the world's largest cities, surrounded by endless and varied things to interest her—reading material, TV programs, museums, parks, neighbors, interesting walks to take, shopping to do, movies to go to and so forth, is so bored and disenchanted that she must overeat to compensate. But a Masai woman who has absolutely nothing to occupy her time except the dull monotony of her daily chores, plus an occasional festival, is never bored and never disenchanted and hence never overeats? Does this sound possible?

Isn't it possible, instead, that the Masai woman stays slim because her daily food nourishes her but does not make her fat, no matter how much of it she eats and how bored she is? And, since she feels well nourished, she feels no need to overeat. Isn't it possible that the New York woman is surrounded on every side with food which is not only immensely fattening, but also so lacking in nourishment that she suffers from a constant, pathological hunger which no amount of coke and doughnuts, pie and candy bars will ever satisfy?

Dr. Stefansson and other explorers who have visited the Eskimos, living as they have lived for ages, tell us that they existed almost entirely on protein and fat with lots of water. Before they were exposed to the white man's beneficent concern which brought them white flour products and sugar, they lived almost entirely on fatty meat and fish. Eskimos were not fat, although their heavy clothing gave them a roly poly appearance. How does this happen?

If we are to believe the psychologists and sociologists, an Eskimo has never suffered from anxiety or stress, has never had the urge to put things into his mouth, has never had any differences of opinion with family or friends which distressed him, has never felt frustrated or bored, lonely or tense. Considering that their lives and ways of making a living were, from time immemorial, probably more difficult than those of any other people on the face of the globe, such generalities are obviously absurd when they are applied to the Eskimos. It is perfectly apparent that "uncivilized" Eskimos stayed lean and fit because they ate food which did not make them fat, no matter how much of it they ate.

It is also a matter of dreary record how soon the good health and the good figures of the Eskimos and of the rural Africans disappear when they are introduced to the inexpensive, attractive, easy-to-chew food of the white man: pasta, white bread, sugar, jams, pastry, candy, soft drinks and the rest.

It would seem worthwhile to insist upon a gigantic experiment being mounted, in which we would find out more about such things, except that the experiments have already been performed and duly recorded. We need look no farther than the state of our own Indian population to see what poverty and a turning to cheap food rich in starch and sugar has done to the health of people who, for all the ages of their existence on this continent, lived on protein and fat, with some unrefined carbohydrate in the form of fruits, nuts, acorns, roots, grasses and grains.

It is apparently easy for sociologists to understand that cigarette advertising, which presents smoking as something infinitely desirable, causes people to smoke. They can understand that car advertising inspires young people especially to worship automobiles almost as people in former times worshipped gods. But it is apparently impossible for most psychologists, psychiatrists or sociologists in the field of obesity control to comprehend that the advertising of food which is fattening without being in any way nourishing has become the greatest propaganda campaign of all time, that it is inescapable wherever you go, even in the pages of many medical journals which long ago stopped carrying ads for liquor and cigarettes.

Obviously business organizations do not spend millions of dollars in advertising campaigns unless they pay off. It is my contention that any blame attached to the average individual who falls prey to this relentless propaganda should be transferred instead to the industry which persuaded him into this trap. The food business is the largest business in America, except for the munitions business. They have more money to spend than any other industry to persuade you that their wares are not only desirable, but delicious; that they will nourish you, keep you slim, make you sexy, brighten your reputation for being a gourmet and a gourmet cook.

The food industry likewise has plenty of money to supply samples for home economics classes, and scholarships, prizes, recipe contests and luxury cruises for student nutritionists and home economics majors. Most magazines and newspapers are supported in large part by food advertising, so a large portion of their pages is taken up with talk about food, pictures of food, extravagant descriptions of food.

The food industry also has money these days to induce prominent university scientists to sell their wares for them. This is one reason why you will find so many articles on diet

179

and overweight written by such experts which counsel you merely to eat less of what you are now eating in order to lose weight. This is well nigh impossible, if you are now living on a diet that contains a lot of refined carbohydrate. You are probably addicted to refined carbohydrate. Telling you to eat less of it is like telling a heroin addict to try taking a little less of his drug every day. *It simply doesn't work*.

And finally, of course, it's our fault that we eat too much. We grew up when the incessant yammer of the radio, the TV, the magazine and newspaper ads screamed at us, hammered at us, badgered, bullied, conned, and inveigled us into trying every new product. And now that the results are disastrous, we are told by sage psychological and sociological seers that it's our fault it all happened. We listened. We did what the multi-billion dollar ad campaigns told us to do. So we're fat, we're unhappy, we're sick and we're faced with a dreary future filled with threats of high blood pressure, diabetes, gall bladder trouble, heart attacks, varicose veins, arthritis, hemorrhoids and many other calamitous disorders, for which we will be chained to drugs and doctors' waiting rooms for the rest of our lives.

And everywhere we are told it's our fault! Why is it our fault? Why can't we be honest and place the blame precisely where it belongs? It belongs right where the blame belongs for many of the other things that are so terribly wrong in our great, rich nation. It belongs squarely on American know-how, American ingenuity and American ability to "conquer nature" and keep it "conquered."

Our vast scientific empire of nutritional egg-heads, and food technologists well endowed with research grants from tax money and commercial enterprises, have discovered how to change foods, make them more efficient than Nature

180

ever made them, make them more attractive, more tasty than Nature ever made them.

"But," I hear you say, "I always have this craving to eat when I'm under stress. When something terrible happens, the first thing I do is open the refrigerator and gobble everything in sight. I just go on eating all day." This is understandable. Unstable blood sugar levels are disrupted in a crisis. You crave food. Stabilize the blood sugar levels and watch the pathological hunger disappear.

Let's say you have some specific times of stress on the near horizon. A difficult cousin is coming to visit for several weeks. It's the busy season at the office which means working late every night. You're probably going to get fired or laid off. You're taking someone you love to the hospital for a major operation. The landlord has raised the rent and you can't find another apartment. *And you are one of those people who eat under stress!* You're bound to put on twenty pounds. Are you?

Open all the cupboard doors and take out all food containing more than five per cent carbohydrate. Lock it up somewhere and mail the key to someone in another city. Now eat whatever you want of what's left in the kitchen and freezer—the meat, eggs, poultry, cheese, fresh leafy vegetables. Eat all you want. Work off all the tension and the stress. Go ahead. You won't eat any more than you should. There are two reasons: it's very hard to overeat when you eat nothing but this kind of food and you are stabilizing blood sugar levels with this kind of food. The pathological hunger will disappear. Try it and see! But don't cheat!

It's not your fault that you are overweight, so just wipe out of your mind all the blame you've been assuming for this tragedy. It's the fault of the people who have been misleading you all these years for their own profit. You can get even with them. Yes, you can. You can do it easily, comfortably and even fairly inexpensively. Just stop buying their products. Walk past them in the supermarket as if they didn't exist. They've had their turn at doing you in and putting the blame on you. Now it's your turn. Ignore them. When the commercial showing the new three-layer chocolate cake mix comes on, turn down the sound, go out in the kitchen and get yourself a piece of cheese and a glass of water. And don't come back until the commercial is over. You could even do a few exercises out there in the kitchen, while you wait.

CHAPTER NINETEEN

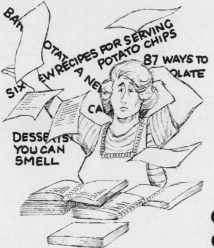

OUR FRENZY OVER FOOD

M*ad* MAGAZINE once had an article (if you can call *Mad's* things "articles") on specialized cookbooks. It began with a *Little Kids' Cook Book* which featured, among other things, "12 Exciting New Ways to Serve Lollipops for Lunch" and "How Much Chocolate Icing for a 10-pound Roast Beef?"

The Teenage Cook Book contained suggestions like this: "The New Between-Meal Snack: Mustard Marshmallow Sundaes" and "How to Stretch 20 Pounds of Candy to Serve Four Guests," "Six New Recipes for Serving Potato Chips as a Main Course."

The Dieters Cook Book gave advice on "101 Taste Tempting Delicious Desserts You Can Smell," "Five Simple Hints for Carving a Grape," "Six Recipes for Preparing One Strand of Spaghetti," "Eat Candy. . . . and Stay Thin—Don't Remove the Cellophane," "How to Select a

Lean Banana," "New Low Calorie Taste Treat: Cream of Boiled Water Soup" and "Eight Sumptuous Meals You Can Make Look Unappetizing and Disgusting So You Won't Want to Eat Them."

Mad, of course, makes ribald fun of whatever is making the biggest advertising headlines on Madison Avenue. And it appears to be cookbooks. A casual *New York Times* cooking article mentions a West Coast couple who own 12,000 cook books. A *New York Times Book Review* mentioned such new volumes as one on making preserves, one by a food editor who deliberately slants her book toward packaged, frozen and canned foods and people who want to cook quickly, a volume just on giving parties, one which is described as "elegant" containing a recipe for a classic French beef dish which contains (in her recipe) quick-cooking tapioca, canned water chestnuts, canned mushrooms, canned potatoes. A salad recipe consists of canned coconut, canned mandarin oranges, canned pineapple, sour cream and marshmallows. Some elegance!

One cookbook appears to have nothing whatsoever to recommend it except that one of the authors is a duke. Then there is a *Wall Street Cook Book* which mixes recipes with financial jargon. There are recipes from every country you ever heard of, cookbooks written in dialect.

Other *Times* ads and reviews have featured such things as a book entirely concerned with the French way to cook anything that comes from a pig, a book of nothing but pasta ($15), a history of eating and drinking through the ages ($16.50), a book on cooking just crab and abalone, one which features only chocolate, another only cookies, another only "flamed foods." There is a cookbook devoted only to ways to use whiskey in cooking.

Full page ads in the women's magazines tell you how to

184

make cookies out of a cake mix! How novel! Or you can make pumpkin pie using any of three or four different mixes, as you wish. Recipe contests lure you into being creative with "convenience foods." That is, you start with a "mix" of some kind and to this unbelievable concoction of watered down and hopped up food, with its ever-present welter of chemicals, you are encouraged to add fattening things: nuts, raisins, icings, chopped marshmallows, candied fruits, wine, sugar, and so forth.

Cooking schools are springing up like mushrooms almost everywhere. These, you understand, have nothing whatsoever to do with nutrition! They are strictly top-drawer affairs where ambassadors' wives and social celebrities gather, at fabulous prices, to learn from the famous cooks who may weigh anywhere up to 300 pounds, just how to make those fabulous dishes, so that, eventually, they, too, can be 300-pounders!

Our advertising industry's obsession with food is carried to such ridiculous lengths that you can hardly pick up a publication on any subject whatsoever without finding at least one article, one column, one page devoted to recipes! Our 10-page local monthly AAA magazine which tells you how to change tires and adjust carburetors always includes a page of recipes—real "gourmet" ones, too, quite as if it were impossible for you to pack for a trip or get your maps together without messing around in the kitchen for a couple of hours stewing up some item of unimaginable mixtures to stuff down your gullet before you start!

The word "gourmet" seems to have taken over. You say that, when what you mean is "food." And by this you mean that you have to add things to the original food with which you started—hysterically, desperately, almost maniacally! There is no such thing any more as just broiling a steak or

185

baking a potato. You simply cannot serve beans with a little melted butter. As surely as you put on the table a plain broiled fillet of fish with nothing, *nothing at all added,* someone will begin to recount Julia Child's latest thing with fish, which takes three hours and involves doing so many things to the poor fish that not a shred of the original nourishment remains in it, and involves also smothering it in twenty-five other ingredients, all of them, presumably, Julia Child's favorite kinds of flavorings, and practically all of them guaranteed to put on weight!

The women's magazines—the whole, slick, gaudy lot of them—are aimed at getting you to eat more. They don't much care how. *Just eat more.* Their advertisers are largely makers of highly processed foods, so their recipes tend, of course, to feature this kind of food. Sometimes you find a recipe for a plain roast beef or a boiled potato. But, why, after all, should any food editor bother much with such things, since everybody already knows how to roast beef and boil potatoes and since the meat and potato industries don't spend much money advertising?

Often whole issues of a women's magazine are devoted to one food—chocolate, let's say, and you are regaled with fifty new ways to use this "taste treat," all of them involving relatively immense amounts of sugar, of course. And the *Mad* recipe for chocolate icing for roast beef seems not so far-fetched, after all, as you leaf through page after page of chocolate-covered everything! You line things with it. You frost things with it. You heap it over the dessert and then over the whipped cream on top of the dessert!

The Christmas issues bulge with fifty or sixty new ways to beat up sugar, flour, butter, eggs, and "mixes" into cookies, cakes, tortes, breakfast "breads" and other delicacies. The cookies mother and grandmother made at Christmas as special treats (years ago Christmas and funerals were about the only times you ever got cookies!) are not good enough for today. Hundreds of new ingredients and "convenience" foods are waiting to help out in your Christmas baking.

Down through the thousands of years that people have been celebrating holidays, the richest and best possible food was always prepared for those days, because during the rest of the year there was not a great deal to eat and little variety in foods. So you splurged on holidays. But what possible meaning is there for spreading out huge feasts of food on modern holidays when the one problem with almost every one of us is that we overeat every single day of the year? Why overeat on Christmas or Thanksgiving?

The splendid women's magazines go right on, month after month, planning parties for you where the one thing that is obligatory is that everyone overeat. They tempt you by picturing the way the Beautiful People give parties, the screen stars, the jet set. They persuade you to indulge your children in ever more and more lavish gatherings where the simple wants of children—a few other kids and toys to jump around with—are snowed under, in a welter of paper caps and expensive favors, lollipops made into amusing gadgets, sundaes heaped with peppermint sticks and chocolate shavings. What child of today, surfeited as he is with sweets, needs this kind of thing to be happy at a party?

And the recipes! Page after page, attractively arranged so you can slip them into your file or paste them in your recipe notebook. Interspersed are ads for such things as cookbooks that feature cakes and frostings made from prepared mixes. In all of these pages the assumption is tacitly made that you cannot greet a friend for a moment's talk without immediately sitting down to coffee and a pastry. You cannot attend

187

a committee meeting, vote at a PTA, talk to Teacher at a school open house, visit the old folks at the nursing home, or stop to get a tire repaired without instantly having to fortify yourself with a piece of cake, pie, doughnut, candy, and a drink of something. Why? Why? Once upon a time there was a reasonable something called hospitality which necessitated offering a traveller something to eat almost as soon as he came into the house. He had travelled by foot, by horse or carriage many tiring, hungry miles. He needed hospitality.

Throughout the women's magazines there are also many articles on the great importance of keeping one's weight down. And the dieting suggestions are endless. Each one is hailed as the final answer. Here it is, girls, how to eat lavishly, and gourmandize on a few sticks of carrots and a few cups of black coffee a day. Dress up your meals, ladies! Add a frilled paper cuff to that lamb chop and you can pretend it's really enough to keep you going until breakfast. Put a dab of artificial whipped cream in your plain bouillon and you'll be content with that for lunch!

Often the diet articles are written by experts in the field of nutrition who spend most of their time debunking "fad diets" and then go on to give their sage counsel, which is always the same—"Eat wisely, by which we mean, eat less. Just cut down on your servings and you're bound to lose weight. Calories do count!"

And on the next page, we start with the full-color chocolate cookbook, featuring 87 delicious ways to serve chocolate at every meal of the day, ladies, from breakfast to late midnight snacks. Eat more chocolate, more—more—more!

I totaled up the food ads in one issue of one of the big women's magazines one day several years ago and found the following:

188

1 full-page ad for salad dressing
1 full-page full-color ad for chocolate frosting
1 full-page ad for a headache remedy
1 full-page full-color ad for candy
1 full-page full-color ad for margarine
1 full-page full-color ad for cigarettes
1 full-page full-color ad for candy
1 full-page full-color ad for oranges
1 full-page full-color ad for margarine
1 full-page full-color ad for soup to be added to other
    dishes
1 full-page full-color ad for mayonnaise
1 full-page full-color ad for margarine
1 full-page ad for a cherry cream cheese pie
1 full-page ad for bacon and sausage

Then among the half and quarter page ads were these:

frozen fruits, rice, corn syrup, mayonnaise, peanuts, evaporated milk (to be made into desserts, of course) frozen pies, candies, gelatin desserts, avocadoes, french fried onions. And a full page color ad for a liquid diet food.

In the editorial copy there were 15 pages of recipes and luscious pictures of the finished dishes: banana splits, apple strudel a la mode, pound cake, chocolate cookies, raisin crumb pie, frosted brownies, gingerbread with red cherry pie topping, cream puffs, frozen eclairs, cheesecake with cherry sauce, apricot mousse, sundaes. Honestly—in just one issue!

One full-page full-color ad in such a magazine brings in

about $40,000. It pays to persuade you to get fat! It pays well.

Today's Health, published by the American Medical Association for the layman, prints sage, stodgy advice on reducing—"Calories do count! You must eat less! You must count calories!" In the center of the magazine is the recipe section, overflowing with full color pictures of luscious dishes. Often these recipes feature desserts. Always they feature sound, nourishing and usually very expensive food, all dollied up with an incredible number of additional ingredients—all of them fattening!

In the March, 1969 issue of *Today's Health,* recipes for meat were featured. A commendable idea indeed. But see what happens to this fine, high-protein food in which there is nothing at all fattening when it is eaten, alone, as meat. With braised brisket of beef you are told to add egg barley, two cups of red wine and ¼ cup of flour. Sauerbraten must contain gingersnaps, sugar, potatoes and bread crumbs. Flank steak is made with two cups of bread crumbs and one-half cup of beer or ginger ale. A recipe for pyramids of beef involves 1½ cans of beer. For meat balls you must add 1 can of pineapple chunks; canned whole apricots go into the veal roast; veal chops cannot be eaten except with two cups of grapes and one cup of wine added. A crown roast of pork you stuff with walnuts and apple syrup in which you use one cup of corn syrup and one cup of red cinnamon candies! Pork chops must be made into a casserole *with six cups of rhubarb, plus one whole cup of sugar and two cups of bread crumbs.* (Rhubarb with pork chops!) Another way to fix pork is to add 20 pitted prunes and one cup of cider, or you can make your pork into a pie with cornstarch and a double crust of pastry.

One simply cannot find any excuse for these recommendations in a magazine supposedly devoted to good health. The only conceivable reason these recipes are printed seems to be that the food editor must fill the pages every month. And they must be filled with recipes no other magazine is featuring. So the cooking gets progressively more and more elaborate and more outlandish with every month.

The dieters' cookbooks seem to me almost as meretricious as the rest. The premise here often is that by making a "gourmet treat" out of your low calorie food, you won't notice that you're still ravenously hungry when you leave the table! You're told that if you spruce up a lamb chop with a bit of parsley and add two mushrooms, you'll be so entranced with the taste-treat that you won't notice the total emptiness of your stomach.

You are advised to eat grapefruit and coffee for breakfast. On your best china plate! For a special treat, broil the grapefruit! For lunch, you won't mind only a half cup of cottage cheese, if you sprinkle paprika on it or cinnamon. To make a gourmet treat out of a lunch of string beans (no butter) add a slice of pimiento, and you have a lunch fit for a king! Do you?

This, it seems to me, is utter nonsense. Your stomach does not recognize a sprinkling of cinnamon as food. Parsley counts in the carbohydrate, vitamin, minerals count only when you serve it by the half pound or so. A lamb chop contains a given amount of protein and fat. You cannot increase it by adding a bit of parsley or water cress, or even a fine china plate. Your body demands food, not fancy arrangements of chinaware or garnishes.

Besides you are told that one reason for today's immense tonnage of overweight is that women just don't have time to prepare meals. So why print cookbooks at all? Why pester somebody already too busy to cook, with directions for

191

boning chickens and broiling tuna fish sandwiches and chopping parsley to sprinkle over everything?

Why not just serve food *as it is* with the least possible amount of cookery? Broil or roast meat and fish. Bake or broil poultry. Pan fry whatever you like that way, liver, perhaps. Eat everything raw that can be eaten that way. This includes all fruits and many vegetables. When you eat foods this way, your tongue knows what it is eating, for human tongues and taste buds and appestats have had millions of years of experience with this kind of food. *You will know when you have enough of this kind of food. You will stop eating. You will not be hungry. And no matter how much you eat of this kind of food, you will not become fat. Nobody ever has.*

I can already hear you complaining. "But I have a reputation as a cook to uphold," you're saying to me, "I'm famous for my chocolate tortes. I always make cinnamon buns for the PTA brunch. And the bridge club counts on my cherry mousse with the whipped cream and the candied violets on top!"

Do they? Well, how about beginning now to educate the bridge club and PTA (especially the PTA) and whoever else you cook these goodies for that there's a better way to eat and it has nothing to do with slaving for hours over a hot stove or making candied violets? How about buying a melon for the next bridge club meeting? You can spend all the time you want shopping in all the markets in town for the best, the very best melon to be had. Then spend all the time you want to spend ripening it until it achieves just the proper texture and sweetness. Then serve it, just the way it is. What's wrong with that?

Why not become the world's greatest expert on meat

cookery, or eggs, or cheese? Why not specialize in chicken dishes, or turkey or duck or guinea hen? Why not specialize in salads? You can literally spend hours searching out greens and watercress—the very best and crispest cucumbers, radishes, bibb lettuce, endive, chicory. Then devise your own salad dressings. If you must uphold your reputation as a great cook, buy all the books on salads you can find. Become famous with a new specialty. Why is it that people insist they cannot give up their great reputations as cooks, when the only things they're famous for are dishes that make you fat?

Or you can become the neighborhood's organic food specialist. All summer and fall your cookouts can feature your succulent organic vegetables, well seasoned with fine salad dressings of oil, lemon and herbs, or cooked sauces. Dream up your own special way of preparing green peppers, cucumbers or snap beans. When you take them fresh and crisp from your own organic garden, there's little you need to do to render them gourmet dishes.

Any well-tended garden always produces far more than you can eat. So specialize in table decorations—heaps of bright red tomatoes, green peppers, yellow squash, with bits of mint or parsley tucked around the edges. Invite your guests to select their choice and make their own salad dressing!

In winter, of course, you can do dreamy things with the food you put in the freezer at the very peak of its sun-drenched goodness. The only added cost is a bit of extra charge on the bill from the power company.

The surprising thing—and really this will be the most surprising thing of all—is the different way you will have of looking at food once you have permanently wiped out of the picture all the gooey desserts and the starchy snacks and pastas. Food—real food—will come to taste ever so much better.

In 1968 a Department of Agriculture survey of eating habits throughout the nation revealed that about half of the families in the United States, rich and poor alike, were not getting the recommended daily amounts of essential nutrients—things like vitamins and minerals. Secretary of Agriculture, Orville Freeman, made a statement which almost—not quite, but almost—put the blame squarely where it belongs. He said, in part, on February 26, 1968, "By all indications emphasis on nutrition education has not kept pace with the increased need for nutrition programs resulting from population growth, *changes in food technology, and the encouraged use of specific food products through promotional activities.*"

CHAPTER TWENTY

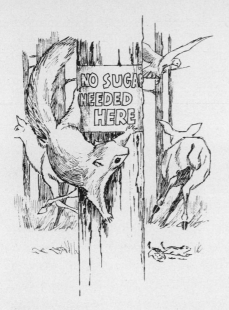

THE SUGAR INDUSTRY SPEAKS

The Sugar Slant is a public relations sheet put out by the sugar industry. In August, 1967 it featured a study by one of the national pollsters on "what people think about sugar and artificial sweeteners—and how they use them."

Here are some thoughts from this little sheet. "In the current pounds-and-inches uproar, guesses have been far more common than answers. Examples: Unsupported news stories announce that over half of the U.S. population is on a diet. Promoters have prophesied that every other bottle of soft drinks will shortly be artificially sweetened. Makers of low calorie foods describe a spurt in production as the dietary wave of the future. The replacement of sugar as our basic sweetener is urged by some, assured by others. Do Americans really accept these claims? And do they act on them? Apparently not.

"For today, thanks to nose-counting and competent questioning, we have at hand a sounder understanding of beliefs and behavior about dieting, diet foods, sugar, family purchasing, calorie-counting and weight control." The article goes on to describe the survey in which 2002 people were questioned about weight and reducing.

How many people were worried about overweight? Forty-four per cent felt that their weight is "just right." Forty-two per cent feel they weigh too much. And 11 per cent consider themselves underweight, according to the pollster.

How should you try to lose weight, was the next question asked. Thirty-six per cent said "eat less." Sixteen per cent of all those queried said one of the following: "see a doctor," "exercise." Other suggestions were "cut down on fattening foods like starches, bread, potatoes, spaghetti, and so forth." Eleven per cent said, "cut down or stay away from sweets."

The people queried were then asked to state which one thing on the following list would do the most toward taking pounds off. Here are the questions, along with the percentage of people who checked each reply:

Cut out between-meal snacks?	50%
Cut out starchy foods?	27%
Cut out sugar and things with sugar in them?	10%
Walk a mile a day?	6%
Cut out alcohol?	5%
Cut out butter?	1%

We are then told that one in ten Americans is now on a diet, and another one in ten goes on a diet from time to time. About ⅔ of these are dieting to reduce weight. The others are on diets essential for health—controlling diabetes and so forth.

Where do people get their diets? The study reveals that

196

52% get their diets from doctors. Thirty-three per cent figure them out for themselves. Eight per cent depend on a friend or relative's advice. Five per cent find one in a newspaper or magazine. Three out of five believe their diets are very successful. The others mostly did "not stay with it."

The survey then went on to find out what people believe about sugar. Or, if you want to put it this way, the sugar industry wanted to find out just how effective all their expensive advertising and public relations campaigns have been all these years.

A bit fewer than three-fourths of those who were surveyed believe that sugar is the best source of quick energy. Over half believe that sugar helps offset exhaustion. The more educated the person who was asked, the surer he was of these two statements! The more poorly educated ones weren't quite so sure.

The subjects were then asked, "Children need the energy of sugar, true or false." Seventy-eight per cent believe that they do. "Is sugar more fattening than other foods?" Fifty-four per cent believe that it is not. According to 70 per cent, a well-balanced diet should include sugar. Sixty-two per cent of all those asked believe that sugar causes tooth decay.

It appears that the advertising and public relations campaigns have paid off very well indeed.

Let's ask these questions a little differently.

Try them on yourself and your family phrased like this. Sugar, as such, was not available to the general public, had seldom been tasted by most of them until perhaps a hundred years ago. At that time, people worked 80 hour weeks at extremely hard physical labor. In all the thousands of years that men have lived on this earth, they have worked desperately hard physically and have had to endure untold hardships. Where did all these millions of people get their energy, since sugar was not readily available? What's your answer?

During all the time that man was evolving and developing up to his present condition, while he was exploring the seas, chopping down the forests, planting the crops, building his own habitations, processing his own food, walking instead of riding, sawing his own firewood, he did not need sugar for energy. Most modern Americans do none of this hard work. They ride instead of walking, they buy completely cooked meals, heat their houses with a touch of a thermostat, do their gardening in a flower pot. Why should such people be told that they need energy that can come only from white sugar? What's your answer?

The average well-planned diet in our time consists, we are told, of a certain percentage of carbohydrate (let's say potatoes, beans, bread), a certain proportion of protein (meat, fish and poultry) and a certain percentage of fat (butter, cream, salad oils). All of the carbohydrate and a large part of the protein are turned into sugar by your digestive processes. What possible reason could there be for adding any more sugar to this, even if, as many people think, one needs sugar for energy? You already *have* the sugar in the carbohydrate, protein and fatty foods! What's your answer to this?

Did you ever come upon a deer in a forest and watch him flash away quicker than an eye can blink? Quick energy is certainly what one would call the way he soars. Did anybody give him a cupful of white sugar that morning? No wild animal has ever tasted white sugar, but the scurry of the squirrel, the flash of the trout or the salmon, the plunge of a hawk, the instant whirr of a pheasant are "quick energy" on a scale that mocks a human being's efforts to move swiftly.

Where do the wild animals get their quick energy since they have no white sugar to eat?

The sugar industry is bent on selling sugar, nothing more. Of this you may be sure. There's nothing wrong with this in the good old American tradition, with the good old American know-how. It's even quite acceptable these days to do as the Sugar Research people have done, which is to question 2000 Americans about how they feel about dieting and sugar and then report the results *almost as if they had scientific validity just because quite a number of people believe them!*

If you asked 2000 people whether the moon is made of green cheese and three-fourths of them said it is, this would surely not constitute a valid scientific finding that the moon is made of green cheese! It might indicate instead that somebody had been conducting a mighty successful campaign to convince people that the moon is made of green cheese.

One result of the survey done by the sugar people was a series of articles—the completely free kind of things that go out to editors all over the country—stuff they can fill up columns with. And editors are grateful for this kind of thing. One of the articles that resulted from the survey tells us "the low-down" on dieting and reducing. "Actually," it says, "most of us are far from feeling that the famous American figure is going the way of all flesh. Despite all the diet talk— and the kooky assumptions about what the dieters among us eat—relatively few Americans are actively on reducing diets at any given time." Why they should say "relatively few" when their own survey revealed that two people in every ten are now, or from time to time, on diets is anybody's guess. Let's call it a euphemism. Two out of ten means relatively few.

"Instead of stampeding us into fad diets, the new nutrition know-how has actually given Americans some pretty firm opinions about the relative importance of dieting and basic foods—including sugar, the best-tasting of all of our foods, and the one that many dieters used to think they had to cut out first." (silly people!)

"For most of today's dieters, weight reduction is best accomplished by cutting out between-meal snacks (recommended by 50% of us) and starchy foods. Only 10% of us think the key to dieting lies in reducing sugar intake . . . nearly every American diet today includes sugar, and some 70% of us believe that no diet can be well-balanced without it."

The article goes on to say that the trend today is to well-balanced diets, steering clear of "fad diets" which may not contain all the nutrients one needs to be healthy. It is not stated, you see, but it is very clearly implied that one cannot possibly have a well-balanced diet without sugar.

You will remember that sugar contains not a single nutritional element except carbohydrate—that is, pure carbohydrate, as pure as if it were a drug. Sugar consists of nothing but empty calories—empty of protein, fat, vitamins, minerals and fiber.

Furthermore, as all independent nutrition spokesmen who are not in some kind of thrall to the sugar industry wisely point out, the more sugar you eat, the less you can eat of nourishing foods.

The average reducing diet—the kind recommended by most physicians—consists of cutting down on calories. The two foods highest in calories are pure fat and pure sugar. The more you eat of both these foods, the more calories you will eat. It is almost impossible for anyone to eat much pure fat. You just don't have any appetite for pounds and pounds of butter or lard by itself, now, do you? But sugar, in the form of hard candy or soft drinks, goes down so easily that you have no difficulty charging up a tab of 500 calories or so in one evening at the movies. One-fourth of a pound of almost any kind of candy comes to almost 500 calories. Ever try to eat a fourth of a pound of butter all by itself, or drink a half cup of salad oil all by itself?

Now let's say you're on a diet of no more than 1000 calories daily. It is extremely difficult to manage such a diet so as to get the daily requirement of protein, fat, vitamins and minerals, no matter how careful you are in selecting food. This is one reason why endless menus accompany any such diet. If you don't have enough meat, poultry, fish, eggs and cheese you will be short on protein, which can get you into very serious trouble, health-wise. If you don't have enough of the bright green and yellow foods, you'll be short on vitamin A—an unhappy prospect, for this involves skin troubles, respiratory troubles, eye troubles. If you slight eggs, meat, leafy vegetables and whole grains you're likely to end up short on B vitamins and iron—another quite serious possibility. And so it goes. Every calorie you spend on sugar, which contains absolutely nothing but carbohydrate means *that many fewer calories you can spend on nourishing foods*. Every piece of candy, every soft drink, every stick of chewing gum on a diet that counts calories is bound to bring you closer to nutritional ruin.

Yet here is the Sugar Research Foundation saying, almost in so many words, that you cannot have a well-balanced diet, even a reducing diet, without sugar! And the only scientific evidence they give for this is the fact that 70 per cent of all the people they interviewed believe this! If you're reading their article rapidly and if you're a sugar addict, as many Americans are, you'll finish it convinced that you have just been told by responsible nutrition experts that you *must* eat sugar to be healthy!

The sugar industry in this country sold 10,245,355 tons of sugar in 1967. That is one reason why the Sugar Research Foundation has enough money to do expensive surveys and hire expensive writers to convince you that there's nothing unhealthy about being fat.

In case you're interested, the soft drink industry, which also deals in a product containing nothing whatsoever of a nutritional nature, did $3,458,632,000 worth of business in 1967. Soft drinks, perhaps more than any other one food item, pose the greatest threat to blood sugar levels. They are usually between-meal drinks, they are cheap, they are everywhere, they don't have to be chewed, they have nothing in the way of fiber to delay their progress through the digestive tract. They hit your glandular blood-sugar regulating apparatus with a supersonic jolt because they contain— many of them—caffeine in addition to sugar. Caffeine, in coffee or any other beverage, seems to have an effect in disrupting blood sugar regulation.

The soft drink companies are blatant in their advertising about how glad they are they have you hooked. TV, radio, magazine and billboard advertising insistently and relentlessly presses home to you the fact that you can't possibly be content with just one bottle of their product—you must have another and another and another. Of course you have to have another soft drink! You have to have another soft drink at about the time your blood sugar begins to rocket down because it's been just so long since you had your last shot of sugar.

In 1966, after twenty-five years of effort, the Mountain of the Food and Drug Administration labored and produced a Mouse: a "standard" for soft drinks. That is, they finally have on file there in Washington a list of ingredients that may be used in soft drinks to the exclusion of everything else. This means that soft drink bottlers do not have to say on their bottles what's in the drink. In case you were thinking all these years that somebody just mixed up a little sugar and water and put some flavoring and carbonation in, you might be interested in what else is permitted in soft drinks. Are you?

Here's the list, published in the *Federal Register,* June 12, 1968. It makes fascinating reading, don't you think?

1. Nutritive sweeteners consisting of the dry or liquid form of sugar, invert sugar, dextrose, corn sirup, glucose sirup, sorbitol or any combination of two or more of these.

2. One or more of the following flavoring ingredients may be added in a carrier consisting of ethyl alcohol, glycerin, or propylene glycol: juices, artificial flavoring. 679 synthetic flavorings are permitted for use in soft drinks.

3. Natural and artificial color additives.

4. One or more of the acidifying agents: acetic acid, adipic acid, citric acid, fumaric acid, lactic acid, malic acid, phosphoric acid or tartaric acid.

5. One or more of the buffering agents consisting of the acetate bicarbonate, chloride citrate, lactate orthophosphate or sulfate salts of calcium, magnesium, potassium or sodium.

6. One or more of the emulsifying, stabilizing or viscosity producing agents: brominated vegetable oils, carob bean gum, glycerol ester of wood rosin, guar gum, gum acacia, gum tragacanth, hydroxylated lecithin, lecithin, methylcellulose, mono-and di-glycerides

of fat-forming fatty acids, pectin, polyglycerol esters of fatty acids, propylene glycol alginate, sodium alginate, sodium carboxymethylcellulose, sodium metaphosphate.

7. One or more of the foaming agents: ammoniated glycyrrhizin, gum ghatti, licorice or glycyrrhiza, yucca, quillaia.

8. Caffeine in an amount not to exceed .02 per cent by weight.

9. Quinine . . . in an amount not to exceed 83 parts per million.

10. One or more of the chemical preservatives: ascorbic acid, benzoic acid, BHA, BHT, calcium disodium, EDTA, erythorbic acid, glucose-oxidase-catalase enzyme, methylparaben or propylparaben, propyl gallate, potassium or sodium benzoate, potassium or sodium bisulfite, potassium or sodium metabisulfite, potassium or sodium sorbate, sorbic acid, sulfur dioxide or tocopherols and in the case of canned soda water stannous chloride not to exceed 11 parts per million. . . . . .

11. The defoaming agent dimethylpolysiloxane in an amount not to exceed 14 parts per million.

And you thought soft drinks were just flavored sugar and water! Does it really seem to be such a hardship to get along without something that contains, or can contain, all the stuff listed above?

The candy industry which uses 1,200,000,000 pounds of sugar annually has announced a new kick—reducing on candy. It seems quite unbelievable but in a fancy promotional leaflet full of words which seem to say something that can't really be said with any truth whatsoever, they tell you that candy has such a powerful influence on the blood sugar level that it can help you in your struggle for weight control! When the blood sugar level is raised, hunger disappears. That's true, of course. And what is equally true is that in a short time hunger reappears again in an agonizing, nerve-wracking way if one has not previously stabilized his blood sugar levels with plenty of protein and a fair amount of fat.

No, the candy industry wants you to eat a piece of candy an hour or so before a meal. This will, they say, decrease your appetite. Or you can eat a piece of candy at the end of a meal instead of "a rich dessert." They do not point out that many overweight prisoners of the candy and sugar trade often eat both candy and a rich dessert at the end of a meal. Nor do they point out that a piece of fruit and an ounce of cheese which may total 150 calories at the end of a meal will go down slowly and be digested as nature meant food to be digested, and will give a feeling of complete satisfaction for hours afterward, because the protein in the cheese will help stabilize blood sugar levels.

Nor do they point out that many addicts can't stop at one piece of candy, especially an hour before meal time, when blood sugar levels are at their lowest, nerves at their jitteriest, tension at its height, fatigue probably at its worst. Why not have two pieces of candy, or three? Blood sugar levels that are raised for a brief time will plunge rapidly and, if dinner should be delayed by an hour or so, we'll be so hungry we'll overeat again—and have another piece of candy at the end of the meal "instead of a rich dessert."

But even more devastating will be the effect if, as the sugar industry wants you to do, you manage to cut your appetite for dinner back to almost nothing by eating a piece of candy before dinner. You will have quenched your hunger with empty calories—no protein, no vitamins, no minerals here. And this will enable you to refuse most of the meat, fish, cheese, vegetables, fruit you are offered for dinner. It just won't work, folks! You *must* have the nutrients in these wholesome foods or you simply can't stay healthy.

Here is a letter from a physician which appeared in the *Lancet,* a British medical journal, April 6, 1963. It tells the painful experience of a sugar addict.

". . . Patterns of overeating vary from person to person. My problem was sugar added to cereals and beverages. To my own concern and that of my wife, I discovered I was consuming over two pounds of sugar a week in this form, and that the amount was rapidly increasing. Part of this was the result of a lifelong 'sweet tooth.' I had always been fond of sweet things because of their taste. But a disturbing feature about my recent craving was that it was increasingly powerful and progressive. If fought, it resulted in most unpleasant symptoms.

"On stopping beverage and cereal sugar, I suffered from sweating, abdominal pain and a liability to syncope (fainting). My mental condition was impaired, and I had headache and subjective head noises. My temper was uncertain. I was continuously apprehensive, and very difficult to live with. These symptoms were immediately relieved by taking sugar. If withdrawal continued, the symptoms settled within two weeks; but it would be disagreeable to repeat the experience.

"In summary, I was eating more and more sugar, and its withdrawal caused the intensely unpleasant symptoms of endogenous hyperinsulinism (low blood sugar). I was caught in a vicious circle. My problem was not excess weight, but a true sugar addiction. The discovery of this

206

fact caused me to revise my psychological attitude. Sugar was now to be regarded as the enemy—always there, always to be guarded against. A brief period of dieting was not enough; I was an addict, and I had to live with my addiction permanently.

"Thinking of this kind is not over-dramatic. It is an entirely practical down-to-earth approach, which, in my case, has removed two stone (28 pounds) of unnecessary weight, and which has proved very useful for my patients with the same complaint. Obesity is produced by many factors, but sugar addiction like mine cannot be rare. In such cases, if my own experience is any guide, telling the patient not to overeat simply produces a tolerant smile.

"But tell the patient he is an addict to sugar, and his reaction will be very different. The very phrase conjures up to him the seriousness of his position, and the necessity for a lengthy and continuous campaign—not to take off his excess poundage but to reorganize his whole mental attitude towards his very real problem."

Most reducing diets today—those recommended by physicians and the writers on nutrition in the newspapers and magazines—allow you some dessert, often at every meal, quite as though you couldn't manage to get through breakfast, even, without a slug of something terribly sweet to keep you going.

As recently as 1952 an expert on obesity said, in *Diseases of Metabolism,* "Desserts are probably made tasty because if they were not so enticing no more would be eaten at that stage of the meal. Desserts have no place in the normal dietary. They should be reserved for a rare indulgence on holidays and birthdays, and for the celebration of other special occasions. . . . . One must not be a food drunk."

Note that he says desserts have no place in the "normal dietary"—that means they should not be eaten *even by people who have no trouble keeping their weight down*. How much less a place should desserts of any kind have in a reducing diet!

CHAPTER TWENTY-ONE

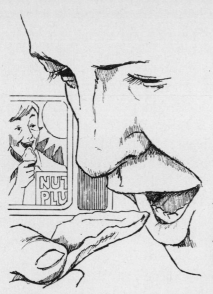

WHY DO AMERICANS EAT THE WAY THEY DO?

Y OU HAVE READ perhaps as many answers to this question
as there are writers and speakers presenting it. It is the
belief of this author that we eat the kind of food we eat—
the kind of food that makes us fat—because there are a
number of very large and powerful companies which make
tidy profits convincing us that these foods are not only tasty,
attractive, delicious, status-giving, but also the most highly
nutritious foods there are. This leads to the only possible
conclusion that we eat too much for the same reasons we
smoke too much, drink too much, and buy too many cars:
Madison Avenue spends billions of dollars every year convincing us that we should.

The December, 1967 issue of *Fortune* gives you a good
idea of what we are talking about. In an article entitled
"The Fight for a Place at the Breakfast Table," Sheldon
Zalaznick lays down the facts on the cereal industry, whose

retail sales totaled 660 million dollars that year. There are, he says, about 66 brands of cereal now in distribution, about 25 of them introduced in the past three years.

There is nothing evil or purposely harmful in the efforts of the cereal people to make you eat their products. Their activities are in the best tradition of smart business practice. They are competing in the best old American way with the best old American know-how, for the cereal business. Their chief victims are children. They spend ninety per cent of their advertising budget on time and talent for TV shows watched mostly by the youngsters. In fact, says this author, the financial success of Cheerios—the second largest seller among cereals—has been possible largely through "the televised efforts of an awesomely stupid moose named Bullwinkle."

So the reason that millions of children eat this particular breakfast cereal has nothing whatsoever to do with whether it is nourishing, whether it is tasty, attractive or even inexpensive or convenient. It has to do with a cartoon moose who is a popular figure with the children. They do what he tells them to do. He tells them to eat this cereal. It's not quite that simple, of course. They believe what the moose tells them because they have been conditioned over the years to accept what advertising personalities have to say. They can be sold willingly.

The pitiful struggles of the cereal industry are outlined graphically in the *Fortune* article. It is disheartening to find that not a single word is said anywhere in the article about the nutritive value of this food, which plays such an important role in the daily menus of American children. From the point of view of the manufacturers and the awesome array of promotion men and advertising agencies who are concerned with these products, they might just as well be flavored cardboard. It never occurs to anybody, apparently, that, if this is the food on which millions of American kids are going to start their day and get along until lunchtime, it better be pretty darn nourishing food. There is actually no evidence anywhere that anybody involved in the whole operation even knows that cereal is supposed to nourish anyone!

A cereal company may spend as much as $100,000 for a drying machine that will mash or puff or cut the cereal bits into various shapes that will seize on the imagination of the toddlers. There are flakes and crispies and pops and bits and chex and loops and crumbles. There are premiums on box tops. Packaging the cereal may involve another $150,000— just for the machinery not the packaging material. Advertising and sales promotion may run into several millions in a few months. Launching a new cereal may thus run into astronomical figures without computing any cost for the actual food itself or whether or not it may contain anything that nourishes.

Teenagers, we are told, are turning away from breakfast cereals. Says the *Fortune* article, "people between fourteen and forty-four years of age, the group that is most indifferent to cereal (in fact, most likely to skip breakfast altogether) now constitute 42 per cent of the population. Rather than lose these former customers, the cereal companies must come up with new products that will appeal to them." There's nothing illegal or immoral about this. It's good business.

The new products are snacks and the new breakfast delight—a tart that can be warmed in a toaster—a new taste treat! We have already, you see, turned breakfast into a dessert-meal. The tart is a cake and the children are sent off to school with a load of sugar in their stomachs and nothing much else. The new products—"cereal-based, jelly-filled" tarts bring in a tidy $45 million dollars a year. Note that the tarts are called "cereal-based." There's still a tiny smidgeon of something related to nourishing food there, most of the rest is sugar.

The snacks seem to be, again, mostly remarkable for their shapes. There are whistles, bugles and daisies, buttons and bows. The snack business is now probably the fastest-growing part of the food industry, according to *Fortune*. So the kids will be attracted to these dainties, will eat them in quantity between meals, with soft drinks. What desire or appetite can be left for real food once you get the kid to the dinner table?

The sugary part of breakfast cereals started way back in 1949 with the introduction of sugar-covered flakes. It's obvious that the more sugar any product contains, the less it can contain, as a whole, of more nourishing nutriment.

Well, the kids have been pouring additional sugar over their cereal for years along with the milk. From 1949 on, the sugar-coated ones added a bit more sugar to every mouthful. You may not realize exactly how much sugar is involved in a sugar-coated cereal. There is no way of knowing even with the well-established brands, since this kind of information apparently is a trade secret. But patents for new processes are filed with the patent office. Recently a patent for a new sugar-coated cereal was filed. The patent calls for a product that is half and half—that is, half cereal and half sugar, or "candy," as the patent calls it. The benefits to the manufacturer were laid out plainly in the patent—the product will keep well on the shelf for many months, the product can be well coated so that it appears crisp and shiny. Nothing is mentioned of the nourishing quality of this product.

Now any cereal food—even whole grain ones—contain a whale of a lot of carbohydrate. Plain puffed rice is almost 90 per cent carbohydrate, about 6 per cent protein. Take such a food and add an equal amount of sugar, which is what is called for in this patent. If at breakfast time the youngsters pour more sugar over this sticky mess the total amount of sugar they are loading into their digestive tract is simply incredible. Yet it must somehow be managed by a glandular set-up equipped over millions of years to handle only very small amounts of diluted sugar well mixed with plenty of protein, vitamins, minerals and, perhaps most important of all—fiber. Today's cereals—almost all of them—are pap. They require no chewing. They melt in your mouth. There is no resemblance here, you see, to the natural foods with which human digestive tracts are accustomed to dealing. Natural sources of sugar are chiefly fruits and vegetables—fibrous, hard to chew, woody even, some of them.

Let's take a look—just a short look—at the relative nourishment of the most popular cereal of all time, corn flakes. This is what one generation of Americans have grown up on. What, actually, does it give them in terms of the things they must have to be healthy and to maintain proper weight?

One ounce of corn flakes, the average serving, contains the following nutriments:

1.6 grams of protein (*the recommended daily amount of protein for growing children ranges from 32 to 85 grams*). Nutritionists believe we should get one-third of this at each meal!

3 milligrams of calcium (*the recommended daily amount of calcium essential for growing children ranges from 800 to 1400 milligrams.*)

.3 milligrams of iron (*the recommended daily amount of iron essential for growing children ranges from 8 to15 milligrams*).

The amounts of other nutrients are so small as to be inconsequential. Perhaps it isn't surprising that, in advertising and promotion, we might as well be speaking of flavored cardboard.. What else can such a food be called? What can such a food contribute to the overall nutrition of a child? When you note that the protein content is almost nil and then remember that the youngster generally heaps several teaspoons of sugar over the cereal, what else is he eating for breakfast but candy—except that it comes under another name?

When you complain of things like this to the people who should be raising a ruckus about this kind of thing—the nutrition experts and the people from the Department of Agriculture, you get the same, tired old answer from all of them. You are told sternly that American people now live chiefly in cities. Their food must be brought to them, you are told, processed and prepared to stay on shelves for an indeterminate period of time. We can no longer have the luxury of eating fresh foods, grains fresh from the mill, fruits fresh from the trees, vegetables fresh from the garden.

What such an answer overlooks, obviously—is meant to overlook, we believe—is the question we asked. What we asked was why do we throw away the most valuable part of our cereal foods and feed our children on the cardboard part? Nobody ever answers this question, because there is no reasonable answer. As you can see from the above review of how cereals are planned and promoted, the actual food value they contain scarcely enters into anybody's consideration for a moment. The cereal industry is concerned with fancy shapes, catchy names, popular TV personalities

214

and competent advertising agencies to manage the whole thing. This is where the answer lies.

Consider the nutritive wealth of that part of the cereal that is thrown away, usually. By this we mean that it is fed to stock animals which of course thrive on it. Compare, for a moment, the nourishment of about ¾ cup of wheat germ with that of one serving of corn flakes. This amount of wheat germ would make a palatable and quite filling breakfast.

The wheat germ provides 30 grams of protein—*all that a very small child would need for an entire day*. It provides 47 milligrams of calcium, 1084 milligrams of phosphorus, 8.9 milligrams of iron (as much as a small child needs in an entire day), enormous amounts of magnesium which is almost entirely absent in corn flakes, plus B vitamins in large quantities. The 1.65 milligram content of thiamine in the wheat germ is far beyond the daily recommended amount of thiamine essential even for adults! There are 17 milligrams of vitamin E in ½ cup of wheat germ. None in corn flakes.

As the organic food movement grows, organically grown wheat germ will undoubtedly become widely available. Whether or not its nutritional content in terms of the above-listed ingredients may be richer than that of commercial wheat germ, there is every reason to believe that the trace mineral riches of this special kind of wheat germ will be much greater—the chromium, for instance, which helps us to use carbohydrates wisely.

So the cereal with which we start our children to school may be just about as nutritious as candy. It is bereft of practically all its protein and natural vitamins and minerals. True, a few B vitamins are restored in some cereals.

In an important article on "Food Chemicals" which appeared in *Chemical and Engineering News,* October, 1966, the associate editor crowed happily that "today on its resplendent colorful shelves, the typical large supermarket carries some 8,000 different food items. Twenty years ago it might have carried only about 1500." He goes on to tell us that one food industry executive predicts that ten years from now the big supermarkets will carry 12,000 items. Half of these will be different from those sold today.

What's wrong with this? The author tells us how it happens, from which we can deduce what's wrong. "Another food company spokesman points out," says he, " 'The marketing of many standard food items—the bread-and-butter items that have been around for years—has by now degenerated into a profitless price squeeze. Therefore food companies simply must make innovations to maintain sales growth!' " So the reason why your children are becoming sugar and starch addicts is simply that the grocery business must make more money and they can't do it by selling you the same old things your ancestors ate—like meat, fish, cheese, vegetables and fruits.

You have to be seduced, somehow, into adding to your supermarket cart every gay, resplendent carton of "new products" which have been introduced with million dollar advertising campaigns. You can depend on it, not a single one of these products was designed primarily to nourish you. It was designed to keep for a long time on the shelf. It was designed to appeal to your eyes, for by now you have been conned into thinking that the bright colors on the box are more important than what's inside. It was designed to persuade you that it is "convenient." Won't take a minute to stir it up, pop it into the oven—and your delicious gourmet meal is ready!

Meanwhile the Madison avenue wheels within wheels grind on. Food editors who write the recipes in the newspapers and magazines you read are invited to champagne parties to taste free samples of the "new product." They get reams of free copy, all ready to toss into the column. What a break! Highly paid chefs in faraway kitchens have worked out all the devices for using the new product in recipes. The editor doesn't even have to check them.

This is how much sour cream you must add to make the thing taste like food. This is how you can stew it up with mushrooms and potato chips, with a lot of buttered crumbs on top. If you like Italian cooking, use the new product in your next batch of lasagna! If you prefer Chinese cookery, just add plenty of white rice to the new product, along with some water chestnuts, and, presto, you'll have a Chinese dish.

In the women's magazines and the big picture magazines, the new product comes out in full color steaming from the crust of a luscious pie, surrounded by the most luxurious and expensive table decorations. You are told in winning prose that this will taste just like mother used to make! It doesn't matter what the product is, you will be encouraged to use it in creamed dishes, in casseroles, in soufflés, in candy, in cookies, in stews—a new culinary world is opening before you! You'll delight your family, amaze your envious friends. Just buy one box—there's a discount for your introductory offer, don't forget!

Where's the trap? What's wrong with inventing new dishes? Why shouldn't we rich Americans luxuriate with any new product our powerful food industry can dream up? Who says we have to get along on meat and vegetables, fruits and nuts?

Nobody does. But if you want to wipe out some of the millions of pounds of lard spread out over the otherwise possibly attractive frames of the American people, somebody has to call a halt somewhere and get us back on the track of eating food rather than a conglomeration dreamed up in a test kitchen. Our tongues, our appestats, our digestive tracts don't know when to say "hold, enough!" when we offer them a new product every week, all gussied up with heaven only knows how much artificial flavors, surfactants, emulsifiers, dyes, maturing agents, firming agents, texturizers, blenders, anti-caking agents and all the rest.

I visited the rather small supermarket at the town near my home, a town of perhaps 5000 people, to see just what desserts were sold there. This is a store with nothing like the capacity of most city markets—a quiet, friendly, sleepy place, where obviously no special effort is made to carry even a representative part of everything that is available on the wholesale market. It is, incidentally, located in part of the country where home cooking is a specialty, where grandma's and great-grandma's recipes for things have been handed down from one generation to the next. So one might assume that, for everybody who buys cakes, pies, cookies or other desserts at the store, there must be eight or ten thrifty housewives who make them at home.

I counted cakes first. There were 25 different kinds of frozen cakes in the freezer. Counting cup cakes, doughnuts and things like strudel and coffee cakes, there were 104 different kinds in packages on shelves. All would presumably be sold that day or the next. There were 68 different kinds of packaged cake mixes which require only the addition of some fluid to be baked. There were 22 kinds of packaged frosting mixes.

There were nine kinds of frozen pies, eight kinds of packaged pies ready to eat. I should have counted the kinds of canned pie fillings and packages of already prepared pie crust mix. It slipped my mind. There were 183 separate and different kinds of packaged cookies, plus several frozen packages and 12 different kinds of frozen cookie dough, ready to bake. There were 24 different kinds of pop-up tarts —the new pastry that you heat in the toaster for breakfast. There were eight entirely different kinds of packaged doughnuts.

Not counting potato chips and pretzels of various kinds, there were 38 different kinds of boxed snacks—of the salted air variety. I did not count the long, long aisle of packaged desserts where you find the puddings of every sort. Just for fun I counted the various kinds of potato products you can buy in this one store, in addition to plain old raw potatoes in their plastic bags. There were 24—dried, puffed, scalloped, mashed, frozen french fried, frozen puffed french fried, and so on.

I stopped at the shelves of canned and bottled baby foods. There is considerable alarm about baby foods among medical men and nutrition researchers whose field is the study of salt and the various things too much salt can do to you in the way of ill health. It seems that the average baby, eating milk and canned baby foods, may consume every day an amount of salt equivalent to 23 grams a day for an adult which is about twice the amount eaten by the average adult American.

Since it is feared that the average adult consumes far more salt than he should have, in relation to the good health of his circulatory system, it seems that the average baby consuming twice as much, relatively speaking, is in the process of becoming a salt addict, due to the relatively enormous amounts of salt present in these prepared baby foods. No baby has any need for added salt, you understand, or even likes the taste of it. The baby foods are salted heavily because mama likes the taste of salt and mama usually tastes them to see whether they are good enough for her child.

So it seems that our processed baby foods may be making circulatory cripples out of our children before they even attain to eating much solid food, for an addiction to salt is a grievously hard thing to overcome, as any adult who has been put on a salt-free diet can tell you.

Nobody seems to be worried about making sugar addicts out of our babies. Everyone seems to think that babies come into the world with a craving for candy which must be catered to on every occasion when you want to win baby's good will. But then, of course, baby gets all that fine prepared baby food, so there is no question of his being well nourished no matter how much candy we feed him, now, is there?

Would it surprise you to know that every jar of baby food I looked at, except those containing meat or poultry, listed sugar among its ingredients? When apricots are prepared for baby, sugar is added, apparently to make them as sweet as they have to be to appeal to his mother's jaded appetite for sugar. Jars of carrots, peas, squash and corn for baby all have sugar added. If you were cooking these vegetables at home you would, we hope, not add sugar. But somehow, once inside a jar they must be well sugared or . . . or what? Is it possible the makers of baby foods believe that babies are born craving sugar?

There seems to be the impression, too, that no baby can possibly be well fed unless he is coaxed into eating all manner of fancy combinations and permutations of puréed food. He can have something called "tropical fruit dessert," or applesauce with cherries in it, just to spruce up the apple taste. He can have cherry vanilla pudding or custard pudding or something called cherry gell. If this is made of the regulation sour cherries that we use for jam, there must be enough sugar in this jar almost to qualify it as candy, for cherries are very sour without lots and lots of sugar.

In most of the "convenience foods" the prepared-for-cooking things or mixes, the list of added chemicals is usually longer than the list of food ingredients, as it would have to be in order to preserve any mixture containing shortening, eggs and other highly perishable items. These things must be manufactured to stand for long periods of time on the shelf, you understand.

And each chemical additive, each synthetic flavoring and chemical dye renders the product just that much farther away from natural food whose subtle flavors and colors are an intimate part of its whole nature. So we can look forward to a time when the kids who are growing up today will refuse to eat a real pineapple. It doesn't have the real pineapple taste that you get in a dessert well spiked with whatever chemical they are using for pineapple taste in that particular product. Here are some of the flavorings that produce the pineapple taste, in case you're interested:

Allyl cyclohexanebutyrate, allyl cyclohexanepropionate, allyl 2-Furoate, allyl hexanoate, allyl phenylacetate, insoamyl cinnamate, isoamyl formate, ... the list goes on and on.

Do you really believe, down in your heart, that a food flavored with these chemicals, and perhaps several hundred more like them, tastes better than a real, live pineapple? The chances are your children and grandchildren will prefer the chemical taste because they have grown up with it and they will come to think of real live food as pallid and uninteresting, compared to the hopped up taste of the chemicals.

When that time comes, what will have happened to their

221

inborn appestat, their ability to choose the foods for which they have inherited a need and a taste down through millions of years of evolution? The nose, the tongue, the taste buds, the inside of the mouth where you roll the food around, the throat down which you swallow it—how will any of these intricately tuned apparatuses be able to make any sense at all of what and how much to eat when their food has taken on a completely synthetic nature having little or nothing to do with real food?

The day is not far off. There are already jars on the supermarket shelf consisting of nothing but chemicals and sugar, masquerading as food on the label, in weasel words which seem to indicate, without quite saying it, that here is a food that is even more nourishing than the real thing!

The giant agricultural industry is developing more and more new varieties of plants which fill some special purpose relating to disease resistance, ease of harvesting, resistance to weather conditions, color, size, shape of fruit and so on, with almost no consideration ever given to either the taste of the final product or its nutritive value.

Square tomatoes won't roll off the shelves where they are being processed. Who cares what they taste like? Strawberry plants which produce their berries all at the same time and at the same height from the ground can be harvested by running a huge machine over the fields. Who cares whether this variety (developed solely for ease of harvesting) has any strawberry taste left?

I have been told by one eminent plant expert that the soil today is considered nothing more than an anchor to hold the plant in the ground. Its worth as a source of nutrients is not considered at all. All the nutrients must come from chemicals!

By the time our grandchildren are grown, there is every

possibility that such foods will be the only ones available. Their taste and nutrient value will be controlled in chemical laboratories which turn out the synthetic vitamin preparations, the dyes, flavorings and thousands of other food chemicals.

Organically grown food, bearing its own sun-and-soil-given nutrients, its own fine flavor and color, will be something strange and exotic. And, chances are, our grandchildren and great-grandchildren will just not like the taste! We must not let such a day come to pass! For then our removal from the soil (which is our beginning) will be complete and irrevocable.

In February, 1968, the Department of Agriculture announced the results of a new survey on the eating habits of Americans. Their experts interviewed 7500 families and recorded their purchases of food over a period of time.

They were alarmed at the findings. The *New York Times,* reporting the survey, headlined the story, "Poor Dietary Habits Called Peril to 20% in a Federal Study." The Department found that one household in every five—twenty per cent of all of us—eats, by the official standard, a nutritionally "poor" diet.

Families in upper income groups were in the "poor" category as well as less affluent groups. *Only half the households queried were eating enough of the right foods to be characterized as a nutritionally "good" diet.* Nobody suggested that anybody was starving or even badly nourished. But, said the Department experts, malnutrition "might result" if these people continue to eat a poor diet for months or years. And, of course, there seems to be every reason to believe that they will.

What are the chief reasons for these bad choices of food among the people, who have to choose from, the best, the

223

handsomest, the most nutritious array of foods ever presented to a nation in all of history? People are using fewer dairy products, said the experts, and fewer fruits and vegetables. And, perhaps more important, they are using more bakery products and 27 per cent more of a category of foods listed as "soups and mixtures."

Bakery products are cakes, doughnuts, cookies, rolls, crackers, french pastries, pies, and all the luscious, tempting goodies spread out fresh or frozen in the bakery department of the supermarket. Mixtures are those attractive boxes which stretch out almost endlessly on the shelves— cake mixes, muffin mixes, icing mixes, cookie mixes, ready to bake cookies, candy mixes, ice cream cones, snacks, sauces, ready to eat dishes like fancy rice and scalloped things for first courses. Carbohydrate, most of it. Furthermore, carbohydrate so mixed and so flavored, so perverted from anything related to grains or vegetables or natural sources of sugar like fruit, that the tongue and the appestat do not know how to deal with such foods. These are the foods of which the American people are eating *27 per cent more than ever before.*

It's not surprising. These are the foods which are being promoted by the costliest advertising campaigns in the history of the world. News and comment about these foods, recipes involving them, testimonials on their tastiness are far more ubiquitous than ads for cigarettes. In addition to being delightful to taste, they are handsomely presented, they make glorious dishes when they are served, their very variety and novelty guarantee the hostess who serves them that her reputation as a gourmet cook will be enhanced.

Conversations go like this. I'm sure you have heard many of them.

"What kind of wonderful goody is this?"

"It's something new."

"Did you make it yourself or is it a mix?"

"It's partly both. First you take the orange cake mix—you know, the one with the red box. You can get it at the Fine-food market. Then you take a package of pastry mix and add some ground almonds. You put the pastry mix into a cake pan and drizzle some canned chocolate sauce over it . . ." and so on and so on. The result is a confection which one might label "instant diabetes." The recipe was in the morning paper. The boxes of mix were all readily and cheaply available a block away at the market. There weren't even any pans to wash, since the mix people generously provided a disposable pan.

The gentleman who spoke for the food chemical industry said, in *Chemical and Engineering News*, October 10, 1966, "The housewife of today, who may very likely have an outside job or be deeply involved in community activities, is no longer willing to spend three hours in the kitchen preparing dinner . . . . she is quite willing to pay the extra price for what food companies elegantly call 'foods with built-in maid service.' . . . Remember, to the housewife reading the ads, just about the most exciting word in the world is NEW."

National health is not important. National overweight in terms of millions of pounds is of no interest to these producers of new products. They control with astronomical advertising budgets almost completely every word about food that is printed in the women's magazines and the flashy slicks. The enormous amount of space devoted to food advertising in the daily papers, along with the home economics columns and the recipe columns, guarantee that the average housewife will be literally overwhelmed with information about these "new products."

At another point in the *Chemical and Engineering News* article, we are regaled again with the old chestnut that people are "demanding" these new foods. Readers have just been told that food companies must provide convenience dishes because the poor housewife has no time to spend— no time at all to spend in the kitchen. Now we are told, same article, same author, same "experts"—"People generally have more leisure time than ever and have developed a marked preference for informal dining. They are spending more time around the television set or in the back yard around the charcoal grill . . . . these trends have rapidly increased the demand for snack foods (pretzels, onion-flavored crackers, bacon-flavored potato chips, cheese dips.)"

Once again, it's the public's fault, you see. The housewife, who is so busy she cannot cook herself, has, at the same time, so much leisure that she demands all kinds of snacks to somehow get her through the boredom of so much everyday leisure time. So she storms the doors of the big food companies, we are led to believe, demanding bacon-flavored potato chips! *She does?* She obviously never heard of bacon-flavored potato chips until some genius in the kitchen of one of the big food companies dreamed up such a thing, the food company "tested it" and the Madison avenue wheels within wheels ground into motion to convince the housewife and the people she feeds that they have "demanded" this product.

The "bacon-flavored" part of the deal probably involves a drop or so of a chemical additive that makes things taste like bacon, but the new bacon-flavored potato chips can be sold for more than plain ones. And the perversion of food has come another step away from a natural, wholesome taste for a food like potatoes. What conceivable resemblance has a bacon-flavored potato chip to anything like this? What gives the tongue and the appestat their clue as to what kind of food this is and how much to eat of it?

Defenders of modern commercial food become grieved and sulky when you criticize their products. Their defense of the highly processed foods which crowd the supermarket shelves these days is that people are now living crowded together in cities. They do not raise their own food any longer. They do not prepare their own food any longer to any great extent. Therefore the food industry has stepped into the breach and provided wonderful foods to nourish us and to prevent starvation. They really seem to want you to believe that we would all starve by next Tuesday, if we didn't have bacon-flavored potato chips!

At the present moment in history, with all the facilities of agriculture in this country and the facilities of the food companies, with all the transportation facilities and the means of refrigeration and cooling rooms to hold foods healthfully, there is no conceivable reason why every person in this country should not be able to buy every day foods almost as fresh as if he had picked them from his own garden, meats almost as fresh as if he had butchered the animal that day himself, fruits ripened on the trees, salad greens picked that morning, whole grain breads and cereals so skillfully ground and stored that they have a taste like the ravishing smell of a grain mill where the fresh grain is being ground.

We could eat like this if we wanted to badly enough. And no matter how big our cities become and how mechanized our agriculture, it would still be possible to provide this kind of food if the public demanded it. But there's not much money to be made selling this kind of food, these days, you see. The money is made in foods like bacon-flavored potato chips. So we are persuaded into believing that this is really what we want to eat. In fact, we are told that we have "demanded" this kind of food.

As the years go by, and generations of kids grow up who have had almost no experience with real food, the battle will be won. Real food will disappear completely. We will be fed artificial food. In fact, the folks deeply involved in such matters are promising completely synthetic foods and nothing else within a frighteningly short time. Why does everybody stand back wringing their hands and contemplating in horror our increasing national tonnage of fat and asking "Why?" *This is why!* We are turning our people into a nation of invalids crippled with heart and artery conditions, diabetes, and the other disorders related directly to diet. And, perhaps even more serious, we are loading our people with mountains of guilt over the whole business of eating, which started out to be a wholly guiltless, wholly pleasurable occupation—remember?

Listen to the conversations of your friends or the people at the next table in a restaurant. "Oh, I shouldn't have that sundae but it looks so good." "Well, just one more pizza. I shouldn't, you know." "You just can't stop eating these snacks! Well, tomorrow I'll make up for it by not eating lunch." "My doctor says absolutely no bread. But these onion-flavored crackers aren't really bread, are they?" "I'll just take a little nibble off the side of your piece of cake." And so on.

Doctors at present—even the ones best-informed on diet and overweight—seem to know very little about the actual preparation of food and what goes into it. What will happen when we finally get the 12,000 different items the food industry has gleefully promised us ten years from now? What will happen to even the best-kept resolutions to eat just a given number of calories? How will you know the number of calories in each serving of 12,000 different food items? How will anybody know, if at present customers are confused and bewildered by the things that surround them today in the supermarket? And what will the results be *then* in terms of health and good nutrition? And overweight.

We are already seeing the results in the Department of Agriculture survey. Half of us are not eating diets that completely nourish us. This is ten per cent more of us badly nourished than the last survey showed ten years ago. What does the Department of Agriculture plan to do about it? Mostly increase their educational programs. That is, with the very limited money at their disposal for this kind of thing, they will continue to send out press releases urging people to eat good diets. By this they mean, eat the four basic food groups,—meat, poultry, fish, eggs, cheese, milk, fruits and vegetables and whole grain or enriched breads and cereals.

What do such announcements mean to people who grow up surrounded by bacon-flavored potato-chips, dessert toppings that you spray out of a can, wholly synthetic breakfast "drinks" that pretend to be fruit juice, puddings that are just powder until you add a little water, snack foods that you can't stop eating because they're mostly air and salt, desserts that come in cans, in bottles, in aerosol cans, in frozen containers, in vending machines?

What meaning do the Department of Agriculture warnings and pleadings have for these millions of folks who have almost completely given up any freedom in choice of foods, but simply load the supermarket cart with whatever looks cheerful and appetizing in a package? Of course, premiums play some part in their choices. A free towel or cup or toy is often the only reason for buying one package rather than another. And unfortunately, fresh meat and fish, fresh poultry and eggs, milk, cheese, fresh fruits and vegetables generally don't come with premiums. In fact, it isn't often you even get free trading stamps for such foods.

But, as the Agriculture survey showed, the nutritional quality of the food we eat decreases in almost direct proportion to its sophistication, if you want to call the prepared foods presently being offered in such quantity in supermarkets "sophisticated."

Obesity and overweight are one form of malnutrition. Had the Department of Agriculture been able to extend their survey, it would have been interesting to see how closely related are obesity and overweight with diets that do not provide enough of all the essential nutrients. Such a survey would be an enormous task on such a scale. But there is a school of thought which claims that people overeat because they crave the vitamins, minerals and other food elements *which are not in the foods they are eating.* So they are forced to eat and eat trying to get enough of these important elements. The Department of Agriculture survey seems to bear this out, since so many of us are eating foods that do not apparently nourish us completely.

To explain this a little further, one could point to a meal of a soft drink, a plate of french fries and a candy bar—a lunch we are told is becoming increasingly common among school children. The total amount of protein would, in such a lunch, be about seven grams, with almost no vitamins and minerals. Because of insatiable hunger for protein, vitamins and minerals missing from such foods, the child would have to go on eating all the rest of the day, one badly chosen food after another. But with a lunch of two big hamburgers (no roll) an 8-ounce glass of milk, a plate of carrot strips and a banana, a child would have approximately the following

230

nutrients, even though the calorie content might be just as high: 42 grams of protein, relatively large amounts of calcium and iron, plus B vitamins in abundance, 18 milligrams of vitamin C and twice the day's requirement of vitamin A!

Scientists all over the world are deeply concerned with what technology is doing to the human environment. Hundreds of conventions and symposiums are held at which vastly important gentlemen in the fields of water pollution, air pollution, radioactive fallout, noise, transportation, city problems, garbage problems, population explosions, and so forth discuss these dilemmas in the most solemn tones. Grave alarm is expressed over the possibly irreparable damage modern man may be doing to himself with the almost uncontrolled burgeoning of fantastic new technologies which are taking hold much too rapidly and too completely for social regulations—"culture," if you will, to keep up with them.

Everywhere the cry among responsible observers is that we must slow things down. We must proceed more cautiously. Most of all, we must create in the general public some informed understanding of what all this technology means to him personally, and how it is bound to change his life, maybe for the better, but perhaps in the long run for the worse. And the general public, which is, generally speaking, not very well informed about these things, is accepting more and more of the fruits of technology which make life apparently more comfortable, more pleasurable, without any clear understanding of what the results may be in the long run.

The one item which is most basic to life and which has suffered perhaps more from modern technology than anything else is food. This is also the subject about which there seems to be the least concern. I don't know why. I rather suspect it is because environmental scientists generally operate in other fields and are just not aware of what is happening in food technology. If they become aware of it, they only know that, when they sit down to meals, they are presented, these days, with a rather different menu from what their grandmothers prepared. But what's wrong with that? Unless they cook themselves, or shop for food—and how many ecologists, physiologists and physicists do this?—they simply don't know that a complete revolution has taken place in modern commercial thinking about food.

Modern food processing companies proudly boast that very soon we will be eating lots and lots of purely synthetic food—that is, food which bears no relation at all to what we have known as food in the past. One example already on the shelves is a breakfast drink, which, according to *Chemical and Engineering News* for March 11, 1968 is "broadly speaking all chemicals." These chemicals have been mixed to resemble orange juice. Skilled technologists have then blended in a "clouding agent" which gives this clear mixture the look of freshly squeezed orange juice. Something called "mouth feel" is also tested. This is to make your mouth feel as if you were actually drinking fresh orange juice.

Now obviously, if Americans were starving and the only way to keep people alive was to feed them artificial food, then of course non-foods like this might become necessary. But American agriculture is flourishing. Transportation of foods is a flourishing business. The citrus industry is flourishing. Americans can buy all the fine, fresh oranges they want most of the year round for quite reasonable prices. Why should they be persuaded to accept a fake food? Why *do* they accept it?

They accept it because they have no way of knowing any

232

better. New things keep popping up on the supermarket shelves every week. Who knows which of them are real foods and which are fakes? Isn't this breakfast drink just the same thing as canned orange juice? Well, how can you tell? It says right here that it contains as much vitamin C as orange juice, and isn't that what we drink orange juice for, the vitamin C? The taste? Well, it's been so long since we had any real orange juice at our house that this tastes like we've begun to feel orange juice should taste. Doesn't it?

Any child who has been raised to like for breakfast a mixture of chemicals, flavored and dyed, "clouded" with chemicals and muddied so that the "mouth feel" is right won't ever know or care what real orange juice tastes like. If, at some future time, he is offered real orange juice, he probably won't like it, for it won't have the hopped up flavor the chemical drink has.

Food technologists do not know and cannot reproduce all the substances that are in fresh oranges. If they did and could, obviously they would. They are persuading you with the customary astronomical advertising budget, that you really *want* this chemical concoction instead. But for millions of years human beings and their ancestors have depended on fruits for certain food elements which their bodies need. These elements just aren't present in fake orange juice any more than real blood is present in a mannikin. Can your physiology get along just as well on chemical fake fruit juice as on the real thing? Who knows? How many generations will it take to find out if, indeed, it will ever be possible?

Air pollution and water pollution, the problems of noise and waste disposal seem to be simple mathematical equations compared to the unbelievably complex situation which has already developed in modern Western countries, in which people simply do not know anything about the food they are eating, how it is prepared, what it contains, or what it may be doing to them. And there seems to be no prospect of ever untangling all the closely intermeshed elements of this situation, so that even the best-intentioned nutrition expert would ever be able to come up with an answer.

What do we mean by a well-intentioned nutrition expert? One, obviously, who has no axes to grind. One who is not employed by a food company. One who is under no obligation to any food company for his education, his job, his research grants. But the food industry, along with other industries, is moving ever more rapidly and skillfully into the ranks of science—nutrition as well as all other sciences. They have all the money they need. They can offer generous inducements to young people interested in nutrition. They can, and do, endow whole college campuses and put up magnificent buildings for nutrition schools. They can and do pick up the tab for conventions and symposia on nutrition where everybody is feted and made to seem important. They publish expensive magazines dedicated to finding out what is best, nutritionally speaking, for all of us.

There is nothing morally wrong with any of this. From the point of view of the food industry it is highly desirable, just as atomic power plants and atomic submarines, supersonic planes and bombers are highly desirable to the people who manufacture them. I am not trying to say here that the food industry consists of scoundrels and fiends who are trying to do in the American people. Not at all. These are undoubtedly lovely people, kind and generous, devoted to their families, intent on making money, sure, but there's nothing wrong with that.

234

What's wrong is that, instead of spending all this available money to grow ever more nutritious food, and to harvest it in such a way that every possible gram and microgram of nutritive element remains in it, and to transport it rapidly and skillfully to people's homes with the least loss of nutritive elements, the food industry has discovered that they can play with technology, as engineers are playing with technology in every other field of endeavor. With the use of very inexpensive chemicals and processes, they can produce something that resembles fresh food. Then they can add certain nutrients—not all the ones they've removed, to be sure—but some of them.

And so whole industries have grown which depend for their continued existence on food technology—*that is, on making food something other than what it is*. There are the flavoring industries, and the folks who make emulsifiers, and thickeners, dyes, and stabilizers, surfactants, maturing agents, buffers, sequestrants, surface active agents, starch modifiers, preservatives.

You've probably never heard of most of these things. You don't use them at home when you prepare food. So obviously they aren't necessary to food. But the food industry uses them to make something different which they call food. And so cleverly have they managed to fill shelves in the supermarket with foods disguised with all these things that somehow the food you prepared at home may not taste just right any longer!

When did you last make home-made ice cream? Try it some day and compare it to the commercial kind. They resemble one another hardly at all. You probably won't be able to coax the younger members of your family into believing it's really ice cream you've just made. Commercial ice cream is so creamy, so rich, it lies languidly on the

235

tongue, it slips softly through the teeth. If you are thinking that you can reproduce this same rich, foamy consistency with plain fresh ice cream and a freezer, forget it. And if you put what's left into the freezer, you'll find that it's full of ice crystals when you get it out later. Nobody will want to eat it. I wrote to the Food and Drug Administration to inquire why home made ice cream kept in a freezer does not have the same consistency as commercial ice cream kept in a freezer. They told me that I could never hope to achieve this at home, since I had no access to all the additives which the ice cream people use to produce this stability in a frozen state.

You might be interested to buy the National Academy of Sciences, National Research Council publication on *Chemicals Used in Food Processing,* publication 1274, and look through it, picking out the names of additives that are permitted for use in ice cream. I did it once and came out with 939. This doesn't mean, of course, that any dish of ice cream contains this many chemicals or anything like this many. It does mean that modern technology has provided this many chemicals which any ice cream manufacturer is free to use in certain specified amounts to play with, if he wishes, to make commercial ice cream into something that home made ice cream can never be, for you simply do not have access to all these additives, even if you wanted to use them.

Now the Department of Agriculture survey shows us clearly that somehow, for some reason, Americans are just not able to deal with the present abundant food supply and come up with meals that nourish them as well as they should be nourished. Secretary Orville Freeman, trying to find some reason for this, said, "By all indications, emphasis on nutrition education has not kept pace with the increased need for nutrition programs resulting from popula-

236

tion growth, changes in food technology and the encouraged use of specific food products through promotional activities." Most people fifty or sixty years ago gardened organically. They knew the cycles of spring, summer, fall, in relation to the rows of vegetables in their gardens and the ripening fruit in their trees. Fertilizer was animal manure and mulch. You killed bugs by picking them off each individual plant with your two hands and by encouraging birds, toads, turtles, ladybugs. Or you turned the geese loose in the vegetable garden to gobble up weeds and bugs.

The idea of soil as nothing more than an anchor to hold plants in the ground would have appalled any gardener 50 years ago as it appalls organic gardeners today. How much of our steadily mounting toll of degenerative diseases, including obesity, do we owe to our almost complete alienation from the soil, which we have now turned over to a crowd of engineers and specialists who regard it as a dead substance, fit only for chemical manipulation?

A friend of mine who began to eat as I recommend in this book because her doctor told her she must reduce, dropped off fifteen pounds in a few months and talked at length about her diet in the office where she works. She found that there was so little knowledge of nutrition that her co-workers feared for her life. "You mean you don't eat desserts at all?" they asked, "No candy? No soda? No doughnuts? Why, you need these things for good health! You just can't get along without them!" One day a girl from another office stopped her in the hall and asked how she had managed to lose so much weight. "I just stopped eating foods that have sugar in them, mostly," my friend said. And the other office worker asked, "But how do you know which foods have sugar in them?"

This was, presumably, a young woman who had been exposed to the usual home economics course in high school.

She had made brownies from brownie mix, muffins from muffin mix, cakes from cake mix, scalloped potatoes from scalloped potato mix, junket from junket mix, gelatin desserts from gelatin mix, puddings from pudding mix. If her doctor had told her to eliminate from her diet all foods that contain sugar she would, I suppose, have had to compile a list of the 8000 items in a supermarket and then ask her doctor to cross off those that contain sugar. And how would the doctor have known?

This earnest and honestly confused young woman went on to ask my friend how soon she planned to "go off the diet" and go back to eating "normally" again. My friend said she planned to eat like this—a high protein diet—for the rest of her life. She liked it. She was never hungry. She felt better than she had for years. Her blood pressure had gone down. And she weighed just what she wanted to weigh.

"But," said the earnest young woman, "if you go on eating like this won't you just waste away to nothing? How do you keep from losing any more weight?"

It had never occurred to her, apparently, that life wasn't just a long series of "going on a diet" and then going off it again, then gaining weight, then going on another diet to lose. She thought, if she thought about it at all, that this was the way people had always lived, and that if you cut out something like desserts—which must be good for you because they taste so good—then you'd waste away to nothing! The basic concept of nutrition—the idea that there are certain food elements that are essential which must be taken in certain amounts—was completely unknown to her!

How is she ever going to find it out, wandering with her little cart through the gaudy, flashy, meretricious aisles of the supermarket?

238

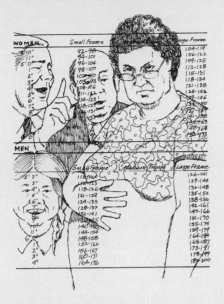

CHAPTER TWENTY-TWO

FACTS AND FIGURES ON FATNESS

WHEN I BEGAN to write this book, it did not seem possible to me that there were literate people alive in modern America—especially overweight people—who do not know the hazards of overweight and obesity, people who cannot recognize overweight in themselves and/or their families. I thought everybody had probably read all the articles I had read about obesity and overweight, had pored over the tables giving average weights and desirable weights, measuring their own weight against the figures given there.

I was troubled to find that, among my friends, many who are overweight do not know that they are overweight, have no idea of what their ideal, desirable weight should be, and express surprised concern when their doctors tell them they must take off some weight because of high blood pressure, disordered blood sugar levels, trouble with varicose veins,

239

hernias, high cholesterol levels or any of the scores of other conditions.

Here are the facts, as they are presented in *Obesity and Health,* a source book for current information for professional health personnel, published by the Public Health Service in Washington, Public Health Service Publication No. 1485.

"A high proportion of our population weighs more than is considered desirable for optimum health. Those persons who are excessively overweight probably are obese also . . . Obese children exhibit many of the characteristics of minority groups—obsessive concern with their condition, passivity, withdrawal, and expectation of rejection. . . .

"The one general difference between the food habits of people who are or are not obese in this country is the fact that the obese tend to overeat in the evening . . . In general, an increase over his desirable weight for height at age 25 if male and age 22 if female is a warning of potential obesity and an indicator that preventive measures should be activated. . . .

"There are no statistics for the general prevalence of overweight and obesity in the total population of the United States although the data available do indicate substantial numbers of obese persons among all age groups. . . .

"The nature of the diet, which in this country tends to be a concentrated source of calories, and the lack of opportunity to exercise in our cities are important elements in the etiology (cause) of obesity . . .

"Contrary to popular opinion, the obese individual is not a repository of nutritional reserves—he may actually be malnourished . . .

"Is obesity a hazard to health? The generally accepted answer is that obesity does create an extra hazard for otherwise healthy people. Weight reduction is desirable for all obese individuals who are otherwise healthy . . . The frequent weight gains and losses indulged in by the many obese patients who practice the 'rhythm method of girth control' may be actually more harmful than maintenance of a steady weight at a high level. . . .

"Recent work on animals suggests that once an animal has become obese it becomes obese more easily and more rapidly a second time. Overweight is at least a contributory or indirect cause of some life-shortening conditions. . . .

"Excessively fat patients have an increased risk in many surgical procedures. Weight reduction in the obese may be indicated before surgical intervention. Obesity is generally considered to be a hazard for pregnant women. Serum (blood) cholesterol levels are elevated during periods of weight gain, thus increasing the risk of deposition (of cholesterol, in arteries and other organs). There is no evidence to show that once cholesterol is deposited it can be removed by weight reduction. It is possible that a patient whose weight has fluctuated up and down a number of times has been subjected to more atherogenic stress than a patient with stable though excessive weight. (Atherogenic stress means potential hardening of the arteries with all the attendant circulatory ills.)

"Unless contraindicated by some specific situation, weight reduction is warranted as part of the therapeutic regime for the obese hypertensive (person with high blood pressure).

"Cardiac enlargement and instances of congestive heart failure attributable to obesity have been reported . . . Obesity increases the risk of skin ulcers in women with varicose veins. Weight reduction has been more successful in obese nondiabetic patients than in obese diabetics al-

241

though it improves the glucose tolerance (condition of blood sugar levels) of the diabetic patients. Obese people frequently have an impaired carbohydrate tolerance that may be of sufficient degree to be classified as diabetes mellitus. Obesity often compounds the physical immobilization that accompanies arthritis.

"Children in many parts of the United States are overweight. Obese children and adolescents are a major reservoir for obesity in adult life. They are more likely to remain obese as adults and to have more difficulty in losing fat and maintaining fat loss than the people who become obese as adults. . . .

"The essential principle to follow in devising good diets for weight maintenance is that the diet should be nutritionally sound and the dieter should not feel too hungry . . . The reducing diet must introduce the patient to a nutritional way of life which will correct a faulty diet pattern and become the foundation for a lifelong weight maintenance diet. . . .

"The person most likely to succeed on a dietary regimen is slightly or moderately overweight, is well adjusted emotionally, became overweight as an adult, never attempted to lose weight previously, and accepts weight reduction as a realistic goal."

Here are some tables. The first tells you what Americans actually weigh—that is, the average weight of the average American. Don't become elated if you find that your weight corresponds to that in the proper column indicated by your height and age. Look instead at the next table which gives your desirable weight.

Here's another table showing the estimated percentage of modern Americans who weigh more than they ideally should. You will note that these appalling figures increase

242

DID YOU EVER SEE A FAT SQUIRREL?

DESIRABLE WEIGHTS FOR MEN AND WOMEN AGED 25 AND OVER[1]
(in pounds according to height and frame, in indoor clothing)

Height		Small Frame	Medium Frame	Large Frame
		MEN		
Feet	Inches			
5	2	112–120	118–129	126–141
5	3	115–123	121–133	129–144
5	4	118–126	124–136	132–148
5	5	121–129	127–139	135–152
5	6	124–133	130–143	138–156
5	7	128–137	134–147	142–161
5	8	132–141	138–152	147–166
5	9	136–145	142–156	151–170
5	10	140–150	146–160	155–174
5	11	144–154	150–165	159–179
6	0	148–158	154–170	164–184
6	1	152–162	158–175	168–189
6	2	156–167	162–180	173–194
6	3	160–171	167–185	178–199
6	4	164–175	172–190	182–204
		WOMEN		
4	10	92–98	96–107	104–119
4	11	94–101	98–110	106–122
5	0	96–104	101–113	109–125
5	1	99–107	104–116	112–128
5	2	102–110	107–119	115–131
5	3	105–113	110–122	118–134
5	4	108–116	113–126	121–138
5	5	111–119	116–130	125–142
5	6	114–123	120–135	129–146
5	7	118–127	124–139	133–150
5	8	122–131	128–143	137–154
5	9	126–135	132–147	141–158
5	10	130–140	136–151	145–163
5	11	134–144	140–155	149–168
6	0	138–148	144–159	153–173

[1] Adapted from Metropolitan Life Insurance Co., New York. New weight standards for men and women. Statistical Bulletin 40:3, Nov.–Dec., 1959 (2)

FACTS AND FIGURES ON FATNESS

PERCENTAGE OF PERSONS DEVIATING FROM BEST WEIGHT [1]

AGE	MEN		WOMEN	
	10–19% above best weight	20% or more above best weight	10–19% above best weight	20% or more above best weight
20–29	19	12	11	12
30–39	28	25	16	25
40–49	28	32	19	40
50–59	29	34	21	46
60–69	28	29	23	45

[1] Adapted from Metropolitan Life Insurance Co., New York. Frequency of overweight and underweight, Statistical Bulletin 41:4, Jan. 1960.

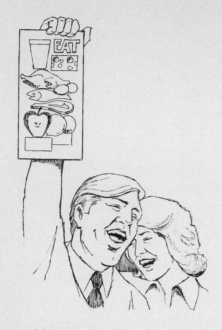

CHAPTER TWENTY-THREE

THE DIET

Dr. Yudkin summarizes his slimming diet in several para-
graphs which surely represent the finest possible recommendations from the nutritional point of view. He says,
"Let me remind you that not only must you eat less carbohydrate, but you must also eat a good diet. For goodness
sake remember that you are very likely to run into trouble
if you try to go one better than the diet and begin to cut
other foods too. Remember that you should have foods
from the basic four twice a day. May I repeat them here:

    Milk and cheese

    Meat (including poultry), fish and eggs

    Fruit, vegetables

    Butter or margarine

"Of these foods, only milk, some fruits, and a very few
vegetables contain enough carbohydrate for them to come

246

into your calculations. . . . You want then, to eat all you need from these four groups. You then eat enough of the carbohydrate-containing foods to give you your carbohydrate allowance. . . . And, finally, you eat as much as you like of the foods which score zero in the carbohydrate table."

How could anyone have any difficulty following such a diet? These are foods which human beings have eaten for hundreds of thousands of years! All that you need to know in addition to this list is the carbohydrate content of the various fruits and vegetables and some cereal foods so that you can take some account of this in planning menus.

As you know, Dr. Cleave believes that you can be guided simply by your own desire for food, if you limit yourself to wholly natural foods. In the case of fruits and vegetables, this would mean entirely raw fruits and berries just as they come from the trees or bushes; vegetables, as many of them raw as possible, the others cooked in the simplest possible way *with nothing added in the way of starch or sugar.*

In all of the diet recommendations designed to regulate blood sugar which are discussed in this book, the only foods limited in any way are desserts, sugar, a few vegetables and fruits that are high in carbohydrate, bread and other starches like pasta, some kinds of fruit juice, coffee, strong tea, soft drinks. Some of the blood sugar-regulating menus permit nuts, presumably because they contain so much protein and fat in addition to their carbohydrate content. For the dedicated reducer, it would seem wise to limit intake of nuts, at least at the beginning.

In *Calories Don't Count,* Dr. Taller forbade all vegetables and fruits and other foods which contain more than 5 grams of carbohydrate per serving but he allowed unlimited amounts of nuts and one slice of gluten bread per meal.

247

Gluten bread is bread very low in carbohydrate and high in protein which is available, so far as I know, only in certain health food stores.

Dr. Gordon of the University of Wisconsin allows any fruits, but permits only small amounts of the high-carbohydrate ones—a sensible idea—only one-half a small banana, one small fig or two dates, two medium sized plums and so on. He allows one to two cups of any of the low carbohydrate vegetables, *none* of the ones that contain large amounts of carbohydrates.

There seems to be considerable leeway, depending possibly on each specialist's observation of how his overweight patients got along, using his diet. *The backbone of each diet, however, is the same:* eat all you want of foods in which the carbohydrate content is zero or almost zero: meat of all kinds, poultry of all kinds, fish and shellfish of all kinds, eggs, milk, cheese, butter, margarine, salad oil, mayonnaise.

So you may plan your meals and snacks around all of these foods and you may eat them in any quantity. You may make them into any kind of "dish" you and your family enjoy, *so long as you do not add to them in the process any starch or sugar*. If you do add it, you must count it in your carbohydrate count for the day, so it's easier just not to add it, isn't it?

Hamburger fixed any way at all is acceptable and you may eat as much as you wish. If you eat it with a roll, if you combine it with spaghetti or noodles, dumplings or crumbs or any other form of bread, cereal, toast or pasta, then you must count the carbohydrate grams in the starch you have added. You may eat any and all cold cuts or luncheon meats in any quantity. No bread unless you count it, and one slice of bread is about 12 grams of carbohydrate. You may eat beef stroganoff, sour cream and all. If you have noodles with it, count! You may have pork and sauerkraut unlimited. No dumplings or potatoes without counting. You may have bacon and eggs, ham and eggs or sausage and eggs, cheese omelet, herb omelet, sour cream omelet, until they come out of your ears, but the first slice of bread or toast, the first muffin, waffle, doughnut or biscuit, the first dish of cereal that accompanies them at breakfast must be counted as carbohydrate grams. So much for the high protein foods.

What about vegetables?

Here are those which contain five or fewer grams of carbohydrate: artichokes, avocados, asparagus, green beans, broccoli, brussels sprouts, cabbage, cauliflower, celery, chicory, chives, cucumbers, eggplant, endive, escarole, fennel, greens of any kind (like beet, dandelion or turnip), kale, kohlrabi, leeks, lettuce of any kind, mushrooms, olives, parsley, peppers, pickles (only the sour ones) spinach, summer squash, tomatoes, turnips, watercress. And of course, things like garlic, horseradish, mustard, soy sauce, tartar sauce, vinegar, which you use in extremely small quantities.

Is it really going to be monotonous and deadly dull eating just about as much as you want of any of these vegetables at any meal of the day? Add butter, margarine, salad oil, as you may wish, to any of these. *But as soon as you add anything in the way of carbohydrate, begin counting.* This means flour, bread or toast, crumbs, sugar. And so on.

When you eat any vegetable with more carbohydrate than the above, count the carbohydrate grams and stay within your daily total. Here are the other vegetables, those which must enter into your daily carbohydrate count: In every case, the count refers to one serving, about ½ to ¾ cup:

249

VEGETABLES	*Grams of carbohydrate*
beans, baked	19–23
beans, kidney	16
beans, lima	19
beets	7
carrots	7
corn, sweet	18–22
cowpeas or blackeye peas	18
lentils	19
okra	6
onions	6
parsnips	15
peas, edible-podded	9
peas	12
peas, split	20
pimentos	6
potatoes, baked	21
boiled	17
pumpkin	8
rhubarb, sugar added	36
rutabagas	8
soybeans	10
squash, winter	10
sweet potatoes	26
vegetarian meat substitutes made of:	
peanuts and soya	13
wheat protein	8
wheat, nuts or peanuts	17
wheat, vegetable oil	5
wheat and soy protein	7–9
water chestnuts	19
yams	23

The same rule applies here: add butter, mayonnaise, salad oil or any sauce which involves things other than starches or sugars. Melted cheese makes a fine sauce for many vegetables. There are all kinds of goodies in the way of herb sauces, mushroom sauces, onion sauces, tomato sauces, vinegar or mustard sauces that can spruce up vegetables, in case you have always thought that vegetables were dull eating. The bright green ones and the bright yellow ones are most valuable to you, nutritionally speaking, because of their vitamin A content. Generally speaking, the bright green ones are, too, the ones that contain most iron, an essential mineral.

The situation with fruits is a bit more difficult. Here is the carbohydrate count of servings of fruits and berries. Remember that "a serving" means a "medium-sized" whole apple, or orange or banana, about ¾ cup of berries and so forth.

FRUITS	*Carbohydrate grams*
apple	14
apricot, fresh	13
dried, ¾ cup	66
banana	22
blackberries	12
blueberries	15
cherries, sour	14
sweet	17
maraschino	29
figs, raw	20
grapefruit	10
grapes	15–17
guavas	15
kumquats	17

251

melons	
cantaloupe	7
casaba	6
honeydew	7
nectarines	17
orange	12
papaya	16
peach	9
pear	15
pineapple	13
plum	17
prunes, dried, uncooked	67
cooked, no sugar	31
raisins, ¾ cup	77
raspberries	14
strawberries	8
tangerine	11
watermelon	6

Nothing very tricky or difficult here except judging the servings. Watermelon, for instance, is usually served in enormous pieces, for no special reason. If you're very fond of this melon, the best idea is probably to cut up a slice some day and weigh out about four ounces, to give yourself some idea of how big a slice will amount to 6, 7, 10, 12 or more carbohydrate grams. Then count, using your own estimate of the size of the portion. The count for cantaloupe and other melons, too, depends on the size of the piece. Just saying ½ melon or ¼ melon doesn't mean much considering the different sizes you may find in your market. And what is a "medium-sized" grapefruit? You simply have to use your judgment about things like this.

And, as Dr. Cleave likes to point out, you can probably

eat all the fruit you want to eat, provided that you really *want* that fruit at that time. After you have become acclimated to your new way of eating, your appestat will tell you when you have had enough, he says. But only if you eat it exactly as it occurs in nature. Juicing it, baking it, cooking it into a pie or a tart makes something entirely different of it.

And speaking of juices, here is the carbohydrate count for them and other beverages. The count is given for 100 grams which is a short one-half cup, a bit less than four ounces.

JUICES	*Carbohydrate grams*
apple juice	12
grapefruit juice, no sugar	10
grape juice, no sugar	16
lemon juice, no sugar	8
lemonade from concentrate	11
lime juice, no sugar	9
limeade from concentrate	11
orange juice	11
pineapple juice, no sugar	13
tangerine juice, no sugar	10
tomato juice	4

MILK PRODUCTS	*Carbohydrate grams*
milk, whole, about ½ cup	5
milk, skim, about ½ cup	5
buttermilk, about ½ cup	5
cream, half and half	4½
cream, light	4⅓
cream, heavy	3
cheese, about ¼ pound	1½ to 3
yogurt, plain, about ½ cup	5

ALCOHOLIC BEVERAGES

beer (8 ounce glass)	8
gin, rum, whiskey, vodka	0
liqueurs (2 ounces)	12–14
wines, sweet (4 ounces)	8
wines, dry (4 ounces)	4

Mixed drinks depend on the amount and kind of mixer. They can go up to 11 grams of carbohydrate for four ounces. Better not mix your drink with anything but water or club soda.

CARBONATED SOFT DRINKS	*Carbohydrate grams in 8 ounces*
club soda	0
quinine water	16
cola	20
cream soda	22
fruit-flavored soda	24
ginger ale	16
root beer	21

Coffee and tea contain no carbohydrate. Most authors of books on dieting appear to believe that everyone in the world drinks coffee at every meal. They seem to force it on you by listing it with every menu and then counselling you what to do about the cream and sugar which they apparently believe everyone must pour into it, in order to make it palatable. If you are accustomed to drinking coffee or strong tea with most meals you would find it wise to cut down at the beginning of your new way of eating, since both these beverages are thought to have quite definite effects on blood sugar patterns. Caffeine, like cigarettes, tends, in the susceptible person, to shoot blood sugar levels up (this explains the "lift" you get), then allow them to plunge below normal, so that you soon begin to feel the need for another "lift."

If you are a coffee or strong tea addict, you may find that you need less and less of these props as your blood sugar levels regulate themselves on the high protein diet. Don't fight it! Don't go on drinking quantities of coffee or tea just because you always have! There is no record anywhere in all of medical history that either of these beverages ever produced anything in the way of good health. There is quite a lot of evidence that they may do quite serious harm in susceptible people. We drink them only because we're accustomed to them and because of the pleasant "lift" they give us.

If you can (fairly painlessly) do without coffee or strong tea altogether, that's the best idea. If you know that you can't succeed at this, along with eliminating some of your favorite foods, then do it gradually. You'll find probably that in a few weeks you won't crave that extra cup of coffee. So skip it! It goes without saying that you will not be using any sugar in your coffee or tea. Cream may be used in moderation. Milk would be a better plan.

If giving up or cutting down on coffee is a real threat to your serenity, how about trying some of the low caffeine kind? If you've tried it and find that it has just no kick to it, why not work into it gradually? Start slipping some decaffeinated coffee in the brew along with less of the regular kind. Harmless enough, indeed, hardly noticeable! Increase the amount of decaffeinated coffee substitute over a couple of months and you'll soon enjoy it just as much as you used to like the caffeine kind. The best solution, I've found, is a filter coffee pot arrangement that filters out those elements of coffee that are supposedly harmful but tasteless, and leaves you just the real stuff. You can make it this way with very little of the caffeine kind and lots of the decaffeinated kind, and nobody—not even the devoutest coffee addict—can tell the difference.

Did you ever try drinking water? It's a remarkable beverage, proven over millions of years to be the most healthful beverage anyone can drink. The wild animals and birds know no other beverage. It assuages their thirst without putting on any weight, without starting any addictive tendencies, without costing them anything. You may remember that Dr. Taller advises his patients to drink a large amount of water every day. He says very positively three glasses of water between one meal and the next. A lot of water. We are told in books about the Eskimos, the ones still eating their original diets consisting chiefly of meat, fat, and fish, that they consume relatively enormous amounts of water, even though they eat no salt whatsoever. It has nothing to do with reducing but a consultant to the Public Health Service recently announced that drinking several glasses of water a day is one of the best ways of preventing and treating respiratory disorders like the common cold.

You may also remember that Dr. Taller told his patients to cut down on salt by not adding any to the food that was served to them. Many reducing diets insist on reducing salt intake. If you are the cook, it would be helpful to cut down on the amount you add in the kitchen as well. There is no physiological reason for us to eat salt, you know. We get plenty of sodium for good health in a mixed diet, and there is much evidence that getting too much can be extremely harmful, especially in certain heart and artery disorders.

There doesn't seem to be any point to listing the dreary figures of the carbohydrate count for all those foods in which it is excessively high. What good will it do you to know that a piece of chocolate cake with chocolate icing contains 68 grams of carbohydrate? Or that only one ounce of corn flakes, sugar-covered and with nutrients added, comes to almost 25 grams of carbohydrate even without sugar that you add? Or that one piece of apple pie contains about 52 carbohydrate grams, depending on the way it was made?

So the best idea is certainly to leave such foods strictly alone. Just don't buy them. Don't make them at home. Concentrate all your culinary skills on preparing high protein foods and those which contain next to no carbohydrate, and preparing them with as little cooking and fussing as possible.

However, some people find it almost impossible to do without bread entirely, even that disgraceful item which passes for bread at American mealtime. And nutrition experts tell us that cereals and grains, generally speaking, do contain nutrients that we need. So here are some figures on the carbohydrate content of some of this class of foods. In general, they follow the same pattern. One average serving contains from about 12 to about 40 grams of carbohydrate.

FOOD	*Carbohydrate grams*
biscuit, 1	17
bread, 1 slice (This includes all variations like bagels, rolls, toast, etc.)	12
cereals, one ounce of cold or one cup of hot	20–25
crackers, 1 saltine (All others have similar carbohydrate counts)	3
doughnuts, 1	16

macaroni, 1 cup	39
muffin, 1	20
noodles, 1 cup	37
pizza (14-inch, cut in 8 pieces) 1 piece	27
rice, 1 cup	41
spaghetti, 1 cup	32
waffle or pancake 1	25

And here is the carbohydrate count on those food items which you may possibly use in recipes or add to high protein foods.

FOOD	*Carbohydrate grams*
powdered skim milk—1 cup	40
1 tablespoon	3
evaporated unsweetened milk— 1 cup	24
flour, all purpose—1 cup	84
1 tablespoon	5
sugar—1 cup	199
1 tablespoon	12
honey—1 tablespoon	17
bouillon cube	0
unflavored gelatin—1 tablespoon (don't confuse this with prepared gelatin dessert which, when prepared, contains about 35 grams of carbohydrate per cup)	0

What are you going to do about soup? Soup is generally served at the beginning of a meal, like fruit juices or fruit cocktail, as an "appetizer." Why do you want an appetizer? Aren't you complaining that you have too much appetite? Why tempt yourself to eat more than you should by taking an appetizer before a meal?

However, if soup is such an important part of your eating patterns that you feel you simply can't do without it, stick to the high protein ones—bouillon chiefly or beef or chicken soup. Skip the noodles, the barley or the rice. Just eat the liquid part of the soup and leave the starchy part in the bowl. You may have as much as you want of the broth part of it. If you can figure out any way to determine the number of carbohydrate grams in the starchy part of any given soup made by you or anyone else, go ahead and figure it. I can't, because obviously the amount of noodles or rice, beans, corn, peas, potatoes or other starchy tidbits in any given soup depends solely on how many the cook threw into it. And every individual cook has his or her own ideas on this subject.

What about synthetic sweeteners? Can you sweeten your coffee with one of the many fake sugars now on the market and stuff yourself with pastries, cookies and candy of the "low calorie" kind? If you have this question in mind you have failed entirely to grasp even an inkling of what this book is about.

Synthetic sweeteners are an invention of the past 50 years or so. They have not been in wide general use until the past 10 years or so. In this book we are talking about the absolute necessity of many thousands of years for humanity to become accustomed to any wholesale general change in the kind of food they eat. Making nonsweet foods taste sweet with an artificial sweetener is pure and simple deception of your appestat, your taste buds, your tongue, your whole metabolic and digestive apparatus. Using synthetic sweeteners is like substituting marijuana for heroin. You're still an addict, but maybe *this* addiction won't be as harmful as your former addiction! *You are trying to learn once again about the taste of real food, remember?* Even a single question in your mind about using synthetic sweeteners indicates more clearly than anything else could your absolute addiction to sugar! You just can't live without that sweet taste? Try it and see! But try it eating only *real* food. Nothing fake.

Finally, remember that your best guarantee of good nutritional health is a wide variety of foods, except for highly processed ones which you are going to skip. We don't know all of the physiological purposes to which different food elements are put. At this stage of the nutritional game, it seems wisest to include everything you can in the way of natural foods. Try all the meats, all the fish, all the poultry available. Don't get stuck using just one or two vegetables and complaining about monotony.

Officially you are told you should get the following, for good health every day: 2 or more servings of meat, poultry, fish or eggs; four or more servings of vegetables and/or fruits, including always one fruit important for its vitamin C content and a dark green or dark yellow vegetable for vitamin A; milk or its equivalent in cheese in these amounts: up to one quart daily for children and more than one quart for teenagers, two or more cups for adults. Four or more servings of cereal foods are officially recommended for their protein, vitamin and mineral content.

This is the way you can look forward to eating once you get your weight stabilized right where you want it. Until then, it is necessary to count carbohydrate grams on the fruits, vegetables and cereal products that contain more than five grams.

260

How many carbohydrate grams are you going to try for, daily? Dr. Yudkin recommends starting with 75, cutting down gradually if you don't lose as much as you want to lose. The low carbohydrate diet that is talked about in so many publications (some of these are listed in the bibliography) recommends 60 grams daily.

Don't think of your low-carbohydrate diet as a chore or a burden. Think of it as a weapon in the science fiction kind of life we are living today. Technology, that mindless, uncontrollable force running along by itself completely beyond the control of human beings, has irreparably damaged a certain portion of our food supply, so that you cannot eat it in more than tiny smidgeons without becoming fat. You will use your low-carbohydrate diet to outwit this force and the people who profit from it. You will use the diet to return, generally speaking, to the unprocessed kind of food your ancient ancestors ate before there was any food technology other than cooking. Think of yourself as an adventurer in space with a new weapon to fight overweight.

BIBLIOGRAPHY

Abrahamson, E. M. and A. W. Pezet, *Body, Mind and Sugar,* Holt, Rinehart and Winston, New York, 1951

Ald, Roy, *Low Carbohydrate Cookbook,* Lancer Books, Inc., 185 Madison Avenue, New York, 1967

Alsop, Joseph, *Drink, Eat and Be Thin,* Signet Books, New American Library, 1301 Avenue of the Americas, New York, 1965

Banting, William, *Letter on Corpulence,* published by the author, London, England, 1865

Bauer, W. W., Editor, *Today's Health Guide,* American Medical Association, Chicago, Illinois, 1965

Chemicals Used In Food Processing, Publication 1274, National Academy of Sciences-National Research Council, Washington, D.C., 1965

Cheraskin, E. and W. M. Ringsdorf and J. W. Clark, *Diet and Disease,* Rodale Press, Emmaus, Pa. 18049, 1970

Cheraskin, E. and W. M. Ringsdorf, *New Hope for Incurable Diseases,* Exposition Press, 50 Jericho Turnpike, Jericho, N.Y. 11753, 1971

Cleave, T. L. and G. D. Campbell, *Diabetes, Coronary Thrombosis*

262

and the Saccharine Disease, The Williams and Wilkins Co., Baltimore, Md., 1966

Cleave, T. L., *Fat Consumption and Coronary Disease,* Philosophical Library, 15 East 40th Street, New York, 1957

Cleave, T. L., *On the Causation of Varicose Veins:* Their prevention and arrest by natural means, Williams and Wilkins Co., Baltimore, Md., 1960

Cleave, T. L., *Peptic Ulcer, A New Approach to Its Causation, Prevention and Arrest,* Williams and Wilkins, Baltimore, Md., 1957

Composition of Foods, Agriculture Handbook No. 8, U.S. Department of Agriculture, Washington, D.C., 1963

Fiore, Evelyn L., *The Low Carbohydrate Diet,* Thomas Nelson and Sons, New York, 1965

Heinz Handbook of Nutrition, McGraw Hill Book Company, New York, 1959

Hoffer, Abram and Humphrey Osmond, *How to Live With Schizophrenia,* University Books, New Hyde Park, N.Y., 1966

Jameson, Gardner and Elliott Williams, *The Drinking Man's Diet,* Cameron and Co., 444 Market St., San Francisco, Cal., 1964

Journal of Schizophrenia, volume 1, no 3, Elias Publications, P.O. Box 3194, Margate, N.J., 08402

Kain, Ida Jean and Mildred B. Gibson, *Stay Slim for Life,* Doubleday and Co., Inc., Garden City, New York, 1966

Mayer, Jean, *Overweight,* Prentice-Hall, Inc., Englewood Cliffs, N.J., 1968. This is extremely difficult reading for the layman.

Obesity and Health, a Source Book of Current Information for Professional Health Personnel, U.S. Department of Health, Education and Welfare, Public Health Service, Division of Chronic Diseases, Heart Disease Control Program, Washington, D.C., 20201, 1966. Available from Superintendent of Documents, Washington, D.C., 20402, 60 cents

Recommended Dietary Allowances, National Academy of Sciences-National Research Council, Washington, D.C., 1968

Sandler, Benjamin P., *How to Prevent Heart Attacks,* Lee Foundation for Nutritional Research, Milwaukee, Wisconsin, 1958

Stefansson, Vilhjalmur, *Discovery,* McGraw-Hill Book Co., New York, 1964. Chapter 34 of this remarkable book tells the story of Stefansson's diet experiments.

Taller, Herman, *Calories Don't Count,* Simon and Schuster, New York City, 1961

White, Philip L. Ed., *Let's Talk About Food,* American Medical Association, Chicago, Ill., 1967

Williams, Roger J., *Biochemical Individuality,* John Wiley and Sons, New York, 1956

Williams, Roger J., *Nutrition Against Disease,* Pitman Publishing Corporation, New York, 1971.

Williams, Roger J., *Nutrition in a Nutshell,* Dolphin Books, Doubleday and Co., Garden City, New York, 1962

Yudkin, John, *The Complete Slimmer,* Macgibbon and Kee, 9 Grape Street, WC 2, London, England, 1964